D1507592

Glamour, Interrupted

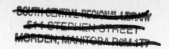

Glamour, Interrupted

How I Became the
Best-Dressed Patient
in Hollywood

Steven Cojocaru

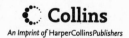

Collins

An Imprint of HarperCollinsPublishers

The names of some individuals have been changed to protect their privacy.

HarperCollins books may be purchased for educational, business, or sales promotional use. For information please write: Special Markets Department, HarperCollins Publishers, 10 East 53rd Street, New York, NY 10022.

FIRST EDITION

Designed by Simon M. Sullivan

Library of Congress Cataloging-in-Publication Data has been applied for.

ISBN 978-0-06-079136-0

07 08 09 10 11 OV/RRD 10 9 8 7 6 5 4 3 2 1

For the true heroines of this story:
my mother Amelia and Abby.

Contents

Contents

Sarah Jessica Parker is inconsolable. Paramedics have rushed in to tran-
quilize a hysterical Jennifer Aniston. Charlize has fainted . . . but that
could just be because her rib-crushing Dior crystal bustier is blocking her
airway passages. Mischa and Demi get mascara touch-ups in between
sobs.

It's my Hollywood memorial service, darling, and it's the social event
of all eternity. Outside the Beverly Hills Hotel, a pale beauty with flaxen
hair wearing a Marni mini and Stella McCartney "tofu" wedges is plead-
ing with the head of security. "But I'm on the list," she says, exasperated.
"Would you check one more time? Paltrow. P-A-L-T-R-O-W."

It's back to back on the steamy sun-soaked red carpet. Renée Zellwe-
ger, in a gunmetal strapless Prada, has "accidentally" stepped on the train
of Halle Berry's aubergine couture mourning gown by Giorgio Armani
Privé. Above the din of shrieking fans, barking photographers, and a
tearful Mary J. Blige serenading the crowd with an a capella version of
"La Vie en Rose," a sign pulled by a small aircraft sums up the general
mood. Up in the sky, it drags a banner: WE'LL MISS YOU, COJO.

By the hotel pool, Bolshoi Ballet dancers in tights and codpieces offer
mimosas and antidepressants to the guests. A Cirque du Soleil troupe
is doing an underwater interpretive dance, a wet homage to moi, en-
titled "Cojó: La Poulet de la Mer." Donatella Versace sweeps in wear-
ing an aqua leather jumpsuit and a mourning veil (from Versace's

upcoming Resort Collection); behind her, her minions roll a portable Thermage skin tightening machine. Dignitaries continue to flood in: Maya Angelou, Queen Paola of Belgium, Queen Latifah, Sir Paul McCartney, Fiona Swarovski, Ralph and Ricky Lauren, and of course, Harvey.

The service hasn't even begun yet, and already the caterers have run out of wasabi-mint crab cakes. Josh Groban is at the piano singing his melancholy heart out, and DJ VICE is setting up his turntables for the post-service dance party. Chairs have been set up around the pool, where Nelson Mandela and Hilary Duff are madly digging through the goodie bags, each one stuffed with a 35cm Black Clemence Hermès Birkin, a Cartier La Doña watch, a lifetime supply of Yves Saint Laurent False Lash Effect mascara, a Chanel bikini made entirely of leaves from Karl Lagerfeld's garden, and a gift certificate from my dentist offering a full set of upper veneers.

In the front row sits my entire entourage: My devoted dermatologist, six hairdressers, three makeup artists, my live-in colorist, personal chef, eyebrow shaper, meditation coach, and my cardio striptease and solar-power yoga instructors. They cling to each other for solace as the celebrities take seats around them.

The music is cued. Bono, clearing his throat, walks to the front of the stage. Julia Roberts shuts off her iPod, Oprah lights a candle, and the whole place goes respectfully silent.

A gong shatters the silence. It's Jennifer Lopez on an elephant, wearing traditional Balinese mourning robes and Graff diamond door-knocker earrings with Burmese rubies. She's followed by a trio of monks banging cymbals and little girls throwing frangipangi petals. "Sorry for being late! Have the eulogies started yet?" she calls out, blowing kisses at the crowd.

She stands on the elephant and balances on one foot, preparing to perform an ancient ritualized Hindu reincarnation dance. Suddenly, the elephant smells a stolen crab cake stuffed in Steven Spielberg's pocket and lunges for it. J. Lo careens backward. She is sent flying and plunges into the pool, her clip-on hair extensions floating on the surface of the water behind her . . .

. . . My eyes open. I am alone in a dingy hospital room, staring blankly at the ceiling. Instead of elegant sobs, all I can hear is the beeping of the heart monitor and the steady drip of the IV. The anesthesia is wearing off and I'm in a foggy state, trying to piece things together, only to come to the horrible realization that my new kidney—after her tragically brief six month stint in my body—has just been removed, along with a chunk of my soul. The raw truth that the surgery of the night before wasn't a dream after all makes my stomach churn.

My body may have rejected the kidney, but my mind is rejecting a future as a prisoner chained to a machine to stay alive. I am facing a future of disease and dialysis. I feel like my life has been carjacked.

Glamour, Interrupted

CHAPTER 1

If My Kidney Had Handles,
It Would Be a Marc Jacobs Bag

Are you wearing eyelash extensions?"
I'm in the middle of one of my signature probing interviews, and sitting across from me is Jude Law and his hypnotically azure orbs. I've already told him that he looks like something out of Old Hollywood, shrieking: "You're the new Errol Flynn, so retro, swashbuckling matinee idol!" But he isn't the slightest bit amused by my interviewing style.

"Um, eyelashes? I don't understand?"

"You have the most beautiful eyelashes I've ever seen," I continue. "I have eyelash *envy*. They can't *possibly* be real: They are the eyelashes of *Aphrodite*."

"I thought we were going to talk about my new movie," Jude says, his face slowly turning red.

"OK—why don't you tell me about your eyelashes in the *movie*, then."

Jude and I are sitting in a suite in the Four Seasons Hotel in Los Angeles, with two cameras trained on our faces. Off-camera, a production assistant is on duty, holding my Gatorade at the ready with a straw in it so that I don't smudge my hydrating lip balm. My T-shirt has been embroidered with a skull of purple antique Austrian crystals left over from the Ottoman Empire. My superskinny jeans are so tight I'm beginning to sound like Jamie Lynn Spears.

But such are the supreme sacrifices one makes when you are Cojo, Professional Featherweight. It is 2004, and my life in Hollywood is fraught with special complications. My personal spray tanner keeps getting called away on emergency because Mariah's elbows have smeared. Linds at the Chateau has stolen my hairdresser, and I'm dying for a blowout. I have to send threats to Will and Jada, warning them that if they don't stop hogging our car detailer, I'm going to put them on my Worst Dressed List.

I think I live a life of high drama, but I have no idea.

When you are a member in good standing of the Professional Gadflies of America Association—PGAA for short—you are bound by strict rules. You must go to at least five parties a week (check). You can't sleep in your own bed for more than ten nights in a row (check). Your tailor is British, your cobbler is Italian, and you fly to Zurich to get your black market sheep-cell face-rejuvenating shots (check).

Growing up in the suburbs of Montreal, I had been a glam-obsessed junior fashionista: I kept my eyes glued to all three channels on our television, devouring every image delivered from the red carpet. It was a parallel universe, and by the age of six or seven I knew the difference between a one-shoulder, a halter and a scoop neck. When I was invited to a friend's house and instructed to "Go play trains with Jeremy," I would instead dart upstairs to the mother's closet hoping to play with yards of carpet-dragging tulle and chiffon.

In Montreal, the most legendary fashion editor was Iona Monahan of the *Montreal Gazette*. The picture on her column showed her in a chignon and oversized glasses for theatrical flair: To me, she was larger than life, and terrifying, sort of a Canuck Anna Wintour. I was writing in my spare time. My English teacher had really encouraged me to develop my talents, and by the age of sixteen, I knew

I wanted to write about fashion. Ms. Monahan was the only game in town, so I cold-called her to introduce myself. I never expected her to answer her own phone, and when she did, with her gruff Lauren Bacall voice, I stammered out how I was Montreal's biggest fashion fan. I suggested that she start covering men's fashion and toiletries. "Why don't I do a survey of local celebrities—radio jocks, sports figures—and ask them their favorite colognes?" I asked.

After concluding that the vast majority of Montreal males enjoyed dousing themselves with Drakkar Noir, a petit career was born. I didn't even have my driver's learning permit, but soon I was writing about fashion and everything glam for a top Canadian fashion magazine. By my early 20s, a raw, primitive version of "Cojo" had emerged, making waves in journalism and hitting every party in Montreal that wasn't canceled due to a snow storm. But I knew that print wouldn't be able to contain me: I was going to be a television talk show superstar, and eventually have my line of hair gels and loofah sponges.

Somehow, accidentally, I segued into doing public relations for the Just For Laughs Comedy festival, where comics from all over the world—especially Hollywood—perform. Through the festival I met a young Hollywood couple, agent Steve Levine and his singer wife Linda. They saw something in me that even I didn't, and kept encouraging me to move to Los Angeles to try my hand at my dream of being on TV. In the early 1990s, to their chagrin, shock, and amazement, I finally did. I packed up my collection of barrettes and moved to Los Angeles, a city whose denizens I just *knew* were panting for the opportunity to hear my opinions on such matters as sequinned sheaths and silky column dresses. I arrived on Steve and Linda's doorstep, and asked them to be my adopted family. Luckily, they didn't slam the door in my face.

The Levines were my shock absorbers. But besides them I was

all alone. I starved, working as a temp at Disney, spritzing Opium cologne at Robinson's May, and working as a personal assistant for a publicist who had me hand-plucking the coarse hair from her chin. I was beginning to realize that my looks could only take me as far as . . . nowhere. Being a trophy boy was probably not in the cards for me. But my Hollywood dream was still alive.

Everything changed when I began to write freelance about celebrity fashion for *People* magazine's "Style Watch" column. "Style Watch" was only half a page and it didn't even have my name on it—I was just a contributor. But eventually I climbed my way up the *People* ladder: As celebrity fashion grew more popular, I was granted a full bylined column.

And then, finally, it happened. I was invited to appear on E!, VH1, and a host of other TV channels to talk about fashion as a representative of the magazine. That led to a regular gig on the *Today* show, as style correspondent and in-house nutjob. I realized right away the magnitude of this: The thought of *me*, being in people's homes first thing in the morning, was mind-boggling. And from the first minute we went on the air, the chemistry between Matt, Katie, and me was palpable. Every time I sat down on the couch with them to do my weekly segment on celebrity fashion, there was crackling energy between us. The banter was so spontaneous: We were all at the top of our game. We never even talked about what we did, or why it worked: it just worked. The mix of the three of us was just right.

In June of 2003, the executives who ran *Entertainment Tonight* approached me, and offered me a job as a full-time correspondent covering the red carpet and doing big-ticket celebrity interviews. The job would take me front-row center, on the front lines of Hollywood. It was the chance of a lifetime. I felt like my professional life had finally fallen into place.

By June 2004, I was flying from Los Angeles to New York and back again every single week: I'd blab about Chanel ballet flats on the *Today* couch and maybe hit a Gucci sample sale in SoHo, and 24 hours later, I'd be dishing with Drew at a Beverly Hills fête. Here I was, and I'd finally achieved my dream of being a television star. I had the heady high fashion Hollywood life I'd always fantasized about: I slept on Pratessi sheets and went to the same energy healer as Ashley Olsen.

But lately, I had been wondering how much of a dream my dream life really was. I was living everywhere and nowhere at all, I barely saw my family anymore, and the only salivating heavy breather who was sharing my California king bed was a five and a half-pound Maltese named Stinky. It was all starting to seem like a big price to pay for the honor of being on Nick Lachey's Top Eight MySpace friend list.

The stress was taking its toll on my body. I'd become a devotee of the Skinny Eastern European Supermodel Diet. I thought food meant drinking a smoothie in the airport or a bag of soy chips consumed while my hair was being blown out in my dressing room, or a flute of complimentary Dom Perignon handed out backstage in the Fashion Week tents. My version of a Hungry Man dinner was a pack of cigarettes, washed down with a six pack of diet soda. I often found myself in a hotel room at midnight asking myself, *Did I eat today?*

My body, which I'd always thought of as being sturdy and indestructible, was beginning to show the strain. My skin was corpse gray. I had dizzy spells. I was running on empty. I began to ask myself, *Is something the matter?* I couldn't help thinking, *Maybe something is really wrong here. Look at you. You are skin and bones, and it's not attractive.*

I started thinking that I should see a doctor. But that on its own was an issue. In the decade or so that I'd lived in Los Angeles, I hadn't seen a doctor once. This medical negligence came despite the fact that I'd always had a nagging health problem: Since my mid-twenties, I'd had elevated blood pressure. But I thought high blood pressure was for old people, and as long as the Sisley moisturizer was keeping the crow's-feet away, I certainly wasn't going to worry about being old and sick.

During the early years, when I was living in a room the size of a Balenciaga clutch and working as a stringer for *People* magazine, I had no money and no insurance, which seemed like a very good excuse to avoid any medical professionals. Then, once my career took off, I simply had no time to waste on going to the doctor. But now, my body was beginning to object to the abuse: It wasn't bouncing back the way it once had. I realized that I was way overdue for a checkup, and finally pulled my head out of the sand. The blood pressure issue was booming louder and louder in my head. Something was nagging and eating away at me: *You need to see a doctor.* Still, it took me almost a year, dozens of red carpets, and at least three Cameron Diaz hair-color switches before I finally dragged myself to see one.

To find my medical sage, I simply looked around for the healthiest person I knew. When I noticed my 88-year-old neighbor doing sprints up our hilly street, I knew I'd found my man. The fact that he wasn't cryogenically frozen yet—that, in fact, he was an octogenarian Vin Diesel—was a good advertisement for his doctor's talents. He gave me the doctor's phone number and invited me for a jog. I declined, but made an appointment with Dr. Goode anyway.

I didn't want the doctor to tell me something that I didn't want to hear: I didn't want to be admonished. But Dr. Goode just asked a lot of questions and wasn't at all judgmental when I told him that I smoked, ate poorly, got no exercise, and had very little sleep. I felt like I was giving him a menu of sloth and gluttony with a sidedish of sin, and he didn't bat an eyelash. I began to relax.

It wasn't until he took my blood pressure that he began to grow concerned. My blood pressure was 200/100. Normal pressure is 120/80.

The doctor shook his head. "This is very high," he said gravely. "Let's do some blood tests." He took a vial of my blood and then sent me home.

I left the doctors office in denial. I didn't take his words too seriously: It was blood pressure. They would fix it. I cut off all signals to my brain and threw my concern out the car window at the corner of Wilshire Boulevard and Doheney Drive.

A few days later, I was rushing from my Baking with Soy cooking class to lunch at The Farm when my BlackBerry rang. "Steven, we got the blood tests back and there were some atypical results. Your kidney function levels are way off. I'm very concerned about them."

Kidneys? *Kidneys?* Did I even *have* kidneys? What did they do? I'd never had kidney problems: My kidneys were clean, probably the only ones in the world filtering milkshakes made of wheatgrass shots and Cle du Peau soothing emulsion. More angry than scared, I threw questions at the doctor like they were punches: "What do you mean? Is it serious? Are you a kidney expert? Where do I get a second opinion?"

He answered my questions and remained calm. "Let's not overreact, we need to take one step at a time. We need you to get an ultrasound."

A foreboding Eastern European nurse did my ultrasound a few days later. The Heifer of Hungary had the thickest ankles I'd ever seen, the body of a Turkish masseur, and all the warmth of a Martha Stewart Christmas card. It didn't seem to matter to her whether I had kidney problems, malaria, or irritable bowel syndrome.

She tossed me a paper gown, threw me down on the table, and slapped ice-cold gel on my stomach. With a yawn, she waved the ultrasound wand over my body. And then, after a quick glance at the monitor, her eyes widened. Suddenly, she wasn't daydreaming anymore. She grew very serious as she waved the wand over my stomach again, and then again, and again. . . .

Then she opened the door, and yelled down the hall in husky Hungarian. A man in a lab coat ran in and stood beside her, nodding as she waved the wand and pointed at the monitor. By this point, I was figuring that I either had the most gorgeous kidneys known to mankind, or else I was a medical miracle, born with a third kidney. But they were still jabbering, and I was starting to sense that whatever was on the monitor was definitely not good. He was pointing, and she was pointing, and they were babbling away in a foreign tongue and finally I couldn't stand it any more.

"What is it? Did you find anything?" I blurted.

The nurse looked down, apparently noticing me for the first time. She said, in broken English, "You speak your doctor."

I was worried, but I didn't want to believe this was something catastrophic. It couldn't be. It didn't fit in with my plans to champion great causes, like going on a hunger strike with Brad and Angie until the Starbucks in Malibu starts recycling their Frappuccino cups. *OK, I thought, something is wrong but it's minor—maybe a benign tumor—and when the doctor calls me, he's going to tell me everything is fine.*

In my dreams, this is how I imagine the doctor telling me I have polycystic kidney disease: First, he orders in tea service from the

Peninsula Hotel, with cucumber sandwiches and strawberry tartlets. He takes a 10 mg Valium—the blue one—and grinds it up with a spice mill with Percocet and Darvocet, and puts it in my Darjeeling tea. Then, he dims the lights and lights a few Diptyque candles. Finally, with a nice soft Norah Jones song playing in the background, and Dr. Phil sitting beside me holding my hand, and with the smell of a fresh leather Hermès tote put under my nose as smelling salts, the doctor very softly says, "Steven, you look stunning. I mean, your outfit today is just so dandy, *GQ* just called and they want to do a ten-page shoot with you. By the way, you have a *little* kidney problem. Not a biggie at all. A tiny tiny tiny little wee nothing kidney problem. Your kidney is sagging and we have to take it out and put a new gorgeous lifted one in. You'll stay at the Four Seasons and there will be just a tiny little procedure, almost like fixing an ingrown toenail. It will be beautiful. There will be an aromatherapist nearby."

That's the way I would have liked it broken to me: gently, without any scary medical terms. But that's not the way it actually happened. This doctor may have been the most sensitive doctor on the planet but as I sat across from him in his office that summer, and heard him say the words "polycystic kidney disease," I felt like I'd been socked in the solar plexus.

"It's a genetic disease," he told me, as I sat there, stunned. "There are fluid-filled cysts in your kidneys that are growing so large that they will eat away at your kidneys until they finally fail. You were born with PKD, but the disease usually doesn't show up until you are in your thirties or forties." Nearly half a million people in the United States have PKD, he explained, and it is the fourth leading cause of kidney failure. In a normal person, the kidneys are the size of small fists. My kidneys were the size of grapefruit.

"From what I can tell from your ultrasound, you are probably going to need a kidney transplant in the near future," he told me.

"But I have two kidneys, don't I?" I asked. "So, if one goes, I still have a good one, right?"

"I'm afraid this condition affects both kidneys," he said. "Both have cysts all over them."

His words had hit my brain and my eardrums, but it hadn't hit my heart yet. It was seeping through my body slowly. *This is a dream*, I thought. *This isn't happening. It's just not happening.*

It just didn't seem real. Often, people who have PKD experience pain in their stomach and back, a result of pressure from oversized kidneys. But the only visible symptom I had of my disease was the high blood pressure. I didn't feel dehydrated, I wasn't in pain.

I pulled it together enough to look the doctor in the eye. "OK," I said. "What do we do next?"

"I want you to see a kidney specialist," he said, "His name is Dr. Moss. Give him a call, and we'll take it from there."

I thanked him and walked like a zombie out to the car. I turned on the ignition, and pulled out into the midday traffic of Beverly Boulevard. Inside me something had died: In my mind, I heard a thud, like something had crashed and broken.

I didn't cry at first. I just drove toward home, thinking about what he had said. I was too numb for fear. The words kept echoing in my head—*I HAVE A DISEASE.* I had to say it again, out loud, to believe it: "I have a disease!" Emotion overtook me, as if I had been knocked over by a wave. I pulled my car over to the side of the street, and I sat behind my steering wheel and wailed.

CHAPTER 2

An Enzyme Kelp Glycolic Oxygenating Facial Can't Cure Everything

I was certain that by the light of day, my kidney disease would have vanished along with the previous night's dreams. My cozy bed, my safe place, would heal me. All my pleading to God—*Let it be over when I wake up*—would work, and the previous day would never have happened.

But I woke up the day after my diagnosis with a sense of dread. My eyes opened and the real world came into focus. There had been no reprieve. My entire body immediately began to ache, from the pit in my stomach to the pounding in my head. The crying I had done the previous day turned out to be the easy part: The shock had been a cushion. *This* was real pain.

I managed to get up and crawl to the bathroom. I had a shoot that day, and I had to collect myself. But I was so lifeless that I looked at my toothbrush, threw it in the sink, and sank to the floor. Everything that the doctor had said disappeared from my brain except for those two ugly words: *kidney transplant.* The weight of these words kept smacking me in the face.

My pooch Stinky came in and curled up with me, but I just lay there, thinking. It was less the proverbial cliché of *why me,* and more of a simple, primal *Why? Why dear God, why now? I'm too young for this to happen! Did I somehow bring this on myself? Have I been an unworthy person?* I felt like crying but I couldn't summon any tears. I rocked back and forth on the floor until I put myself in a trance. The words—adjectives, questions, worries—disappeared. My mind was blank. All that was left was pain seeping through every cell in my body like strychnine.

After an hour, my haze began to clear and I stood up. I looked at myself in the mirror, and my heart fell: I had so much tenderness for the person I saw. He wasn't the firecracker on the red carpet with a microphone: This creature before me was just a child, a very wounded and afraid little boy. *You poor baby* I thought. *I'm so sorry for you.*

I splashed my face with cold water. I went through the motions of showering and getting ready to face the world. The sun was beaming down on Los Angeles with its brilliant light, but inside my house it was like a funeral parlor. Physically it felt like so much effort just to move, as if my legs were lead.

As I headed out the door, I felt emotional numbness beginning to creep over me, as if I was slowly freezing over. I had no choice but to bury my feelings: The fact that I was falling apart had to be put on hold. There was work to be done. It was as if I'd put yellow police tape around my feelings that said, SCENE OF AN EMOTIONAL MASSACRE. KEEP OUT.

By noon, the numbness had grown into fierce denial. And denial was comfortable, like wrapping myself in a fluffy white bathrobe. It was easier to keep reality out, to act as if nothing was wrong, until I reached a point where even *I* believed that disease hadn't rung my doorbell.

I did what any of my favorite celluloid divas might do: I covered up my pain with concealer and industrial-strength waterproof mascara. I went out to do my television interview. And for the next few months I hid the scarlet letter D for disease underneath my designer glad rags, and didn't tell a soul that I might be dying.

Some people self-medicate with Scotch on the rocks: My elixir for pain is classic Hollywood movies. I fell in love with them as a child, swept up in the high drama and even higher glamour. It was pretty heady for an eight-year-old to know what words like "chiffon" and "silk charmeuse" meant—even if my classmates didn't appreciate my use of the phrase "ermine stole" in playground conversation.

One of the jewels of my DVD library is the revered *Camille*, starring Greta Garbo as a Parisian courtesan who is secretly dying of consumption. Garbo made illness look so chic: She was brave and noble because she kept her illness a secret in order to protect her loved ones. As the days passed, and I stayed in the disease closet— not telling my loved ones my own dark secret—I began to think of myself as the heroine of my own version of *Camille*. When you are in the kind of mind-set I was in, your brain travels to dark corners. In a sick way, to entertain myself, I fantasized about my death scene: I was Garbo, with incredible lighting, in a beautiful peignoir, lying on my deathbed on satin sheets, attended by my devoted maid and Robert Taylor.

I had decided that if I didn't say the words kidney disease out loud, it wouldn't be true. Instead, I would go about my life in the usual way. Nothing would change. I wouldn't be a sick person. And, like Camille, I was also terrified that telling the truth would cause mortal pain to the people around me—especially my mother.

My parents, Benjamin and Amelia Cojocaru, are survivors. As children in Romania, they lived through the Holocaust (my grandfather was in a labor camp), emigrated to Israel and then to Canada, worked in sweatshops, and eventually managed to raise a family in Montreal. Even though they've soldiered through hell and back, I've always thought of them as incredibly sensitive, high-strung people. After all, we come from a long line of melodramatic, hot-blooded, emotional Eastern Europeans: If there was Kabuki theater in Romania, my relatives would be in it. Everything was always heightened in our house:

When I was ten years old, my uncle in Israel died—my mother's sister's husband, a man my mom absolutely adored. My aunt pierced the silence of our sleep by calling at five in the morning to tell us that he had passed away. When my mother heard the news, she imploded. There was shrieking, blood-curdling yells, hysterics. She physically hurled herself against the walls, and slammed her fists against the floor. It was single-handedly the most terrifying moment of my childhood.

If that was how she reacted to the death of someone who wasn't even a blood relative, I could only imagine what might happen if she found out that her beloved son—her little prince!—had a life-threatening disease. Revealing my diagnosis would be like putting a knife through her heart. I thought that the magnitude of this tragedy was so great that she wouldn't be able to cope with it. My parents were elderly now, they lived for their children—perfect son and perfect daughter (my older sister Alisa)—they had worked their fingers to the bone to have some peace in their retirement, and here I was about to tell them that their son needed a kidney transplant. These were supposed to be their golden years, a time of serenity, a time to get tipsy on mango mai tai's at the Hilton Hawaiian Village. Instead, after everything they'd been through in their lives, it had come to this? It seemed like a cruel twist of fate.

In August, not long after I was diagnosed, I went home to Montreal for a previously scheduled family visit. At my parent's house, all issues are discussed, bickered about, and solved at the vast black lacquered, faux-Asian, dining room-table-cum-family court. This visit was no different. My mother put out a spread of homemade desserts—almond cake, cheesecake, honeycake, sponge cake, and a chocolate torte—and we sat around the table, catching up.

"My son! Mr. Hollywood. Don't they have hairdressers in Hollywood?" my dad said.

My mom chimed in. "You look like a girl! Can't you get a nice clean haircut, like George Clooney?"

Alisa tugged at my sleeve. "Oh my gawd! What kind of jacket is this? It's *stunning!* When you don't need it, give it to me!"

My sister Alisa knows how to work my nerves, but together we partner in rolling our eyes at our over-the-top family. We take the foibles of our highly-strung parents with a grain of salt and good humor. This is our bond.

But the glue of our relationship is not having the same eyes and gorgeous poufy lips; it's our passion for accessories. My sister may dress like a walking Britney music video—to the horror of myself and my parents—but an oversize Chanel bag completes her . . . just as it does me.

"It's Dior Homme," I said, pulling away from my sister's grasping, vermillion-painted claws. "And don't touch it until you've sterilized those fingers."

"Fancy!" my dad said, reaching for a second helping of honeycake. "How much?"

"Around five hundred," I muttered.

"Are you crazy? What? Five hundred? I wouldn't give two Romanian *lei* for that. I used to support three families on that. After your grandfather's stroke, who do you think paid the bills?"

"Oh no, not this saga again." I rolled my eyes, looked at Alisa, and we erupted into giggles. My family fit comfortably: Trivial annoyances aside, we were a solid, loving family. I looked around at their dancing eyes, so elated that the prodigal son had returned home, light and upbeat. But inside, I knew that I was a fraud: I needed to tell them what was really going on with me.

It physically hurt to talk to them. I needed them so badly that I wanted to curl up into a fetal position and cry, "Solve this for me! Cure me! Make me better! Take it away!" I knew that I should let them in, but I didn't have the courage. I didn't want to shatter this moment and bring them pain. The truth was that I was a wimp who couldn't deal with telling them.

Instead, I began to choke up. "Excuse me," I said, and bolted up from the table, trailing cake crumbs behind me. I ran to the bathroom and barely managed to shut the door before the waterworks started. I felt so sorry for my loved ones in the other room, whose lives were very soon going to be torn to bits. It killed me. I sat there in the bathroom, looking at myself, seeing disease in my eyes and thinking, *This is too much.* But I took a deep breath, came out of the bathroom, and put my happy face on.

And I sealed my mouth shut. In the months that followed, I failed to tell my parents my diagnosis at least a dozen times. I also didn't tell my friends or my coworkers, but for a very different reason: Sick doesn't play in Hollywood. Illness is never bathed in good lighting; it doesn't get its own trailer on the movie set. Just like aging is not acceptable, disease won't get you a reservation at The Grill. It's too real, too raw . . . It's a downer, man.

I was afraid that once I confessed, Hollywood would never look at me the same way again. I have a million BFFs in Hollywood, but our friendships are very one-note, based on the following exchange: I'll say, "You look fabulous." And then they'll say, "No, *you* look fabulous." Then I'll add, "Your hair! My God! Who is doing your color?"

And they'll say, "Oh! *Your* hair! It's so perfect flowy, very London '68. Do you have a new hairstylist?" And then, "That bag! . . ."

Cardboard cutout friendships are the currency of Hollywood. It's all performance. The schmoozing and pumped-up camaraderie are just business: It's all part of a certain language, a certain social dynamic. So you don't expect anybody to care. I was convinced people would treat me like I had the plague. As they would say in polite company at a table on the Terrace at the Hotel Bel Air, my situation was "unpleasant"—a Hollywood euphemism for anything yucky, smelly, grotesque, or unattractive. If I went public with my disease, would the A-list turn its back on me? Would I be completely abandoned? I couldn't face that. I was terrified that my career was over.

Instead, I went back to my frivolous life as if I didn't have a care in the world, commuting to New York and going on live television to feast on celebrities' fashion faux pas. Being on camera and laughing with all 750 of my teeth was the best medicine: It saved me. During those minutes when I was in the glow of the television lights, I didn't have bum kidneys. I was kooky, happy-go-lucky Cojo.

I was so deeply in denial that I also wasn't doing a thing to address my disease. It was September, and I still hadn't called the kidney specialist my doctor had referred me to: In fact, I hadn't spoken to Dr. Goode at all since our meeting that summer. I had intentionally kept myself clueless about PKD: Information was just a click away on the Internet, but I preferred to stay in the dark. A lot of people want to learn all they can about their disease, and doctors recommend that you educate yourself, but I was roundly ignoring that advice. I didn't want to know how badly my body was being beaten; I didn't want to know how quickly it was deteriorating. The gruesome details seemed too depressing.

But increasingly, there was a voice inside that was pestering me.

No matter how hard this is, it admonished me, *you have got to get out of this denial.* Wake up! *You're gravely ill! You need a new kidney, or one of these days you are going to collapse, maybe on live television. Steven, you need care. Maybe they can do something.*

As the months passed, my numbness began to melt away. My romantic vision of noble silent suffering a la Garbo wasn't working out. The truth was that, despite all my best efforts to freeze it out, my disease *was* eating away at me all day long, tearing away at my interior lining. That internal voice of warning was getting too loud to ignore. I began to slowly realize that it was self-destructive not to see a doctor, and the longer I waited, the crazier it was.

I began to notice strange physical symptoms. There were traces of blood in my urine. I would wake up in the middle of the night with horrible cramps in my feet. And no matter how much sleep I got, I was tired all the time—once I caught myself almost falling asleep behind the wheel of my car during rush hour. My body wasn't listening to my mind's staunch commands to ignore the enemy incursion: It was insisting that I take the plunge and call a doctor.

That fall, I finally picked up the phone to call the kidney specialist that my doctor had recommended. I had bought as much time as I could afford. This was the moment of reckoning.

"You are very late in the game," the kidney specialist, Dr. Moss, gravely intoned, the first time I met with him. "Your kidney function is dangerously low. Maybe, if you are lucky, you have six or eight months, tops, before your kidneys fail. I wouldn't bet on a year."

It was as if I'd been thrown naked into the Arctic Sea. Suddenly I thought I could feel my rotting kidneys for the very first time. "What would happen if I don't get a kidney by then?"

"You are looking at two possible scenarios," he said. I was either going to have to get a kidney transplant immediately, or, once my kidneys began to go, I would need to go on dialysis. Dialysis is a life support procedure that filters waste from your blood and excess fluid from your body when your kidneys can no longer do it themselves: I could spend the rest of my life hooked up to a machine.

Dr. Moss promptly put me on medication: I was anemic. He talked about low white blood cells, iron deficiencies, calcium supplements, potassium levels. He stabbed me with needles. He took blood tests and urine samples galore. He told me to make an appointment at the kidney transplant clinic at Cedars-Sinai Medical Center in West Hollywood, immediately.

I had entered Kidneyland. I was officially a patient now. Somehow, I had managed to walk through a door: WELCOME TO THE WORLD OF SICKNESS. We have air-conditioning and HBO.

CHAPTER 3

Welcome to Hotel Cedars-Sinai

A t most hospitals in America, you wouldn't find paparazzi and movie stars hanging around the triage tables, but Cedars-Sinai is not your average hospital. At Cedars, valet parking is practically included in the bill and filet mignon is served instead of lime jello. This is where Britney Spears has her epidurals administered, Lindsay Lohan recovers from "exhaustion," and Brad Pitt is treated for obscure exotic viruses. It is, in a word, *The* Hollywood Hospital.

And I imagined myself as its latest megastar patient. I had deluded myself into believing that my very presence at Cedars-Sinai would create nothing short of pandemonium. On the way to the hospital, I built up my own self-importance in my head until I was convinced I was Madonna and that I would need a disguise to hide from the paparazzi. I had visions of a beekeepers hat, seven veils and a feathered mask worthy of the Venetian Ball dancing through my head. I could practically hear the buzz about my presence tearing through Cedars-Sinai, the gossip bouncing from nurses station to nurses station, spreading like a conjuctivitus plague in a preschool. The rumor would bounce through gynecology, rev past urology, veer right at geriatrics, and torpedo its way straight toward nephrectomy.

I darted through the hospital on my way to the kidney clinic with the collar of my McQueen leather trench coat turned up, hidden behind humongous black sunglasses, anticipating the throngs of stalkarazzi with 300 mm telephoto lenses around every corner. No one was there, of course. But imagining myself as the first lady of Malawi was simply a distracting fantasy, a way to forget what I was really here to do.

But in all seriousness, secrecy *was* important to me at that moment. I was terrified that news of my illness would end up in the media, maybe even meriting a column inch in *Women's Wear Daily*. I still hadn't told any of my family or friends about my illness. I was still just taking baby steps with accepting my plight—and I certainly didn't want them to learn about it from seeing it on TV.

This maiden visit to the kidney clinic was my first foray as a sick person in public since I'd been diagnosed. When I walked into the waiting room, I was still absolutely horrified. There were curious eyeballs everywhere. I felt, surely everyone in the room knew my white blood cell count, my sperm count, the exact size and shape of my kidneys, and my urine output.

Even without the fear of exposure, I was on the verge of a panic attack: Today was the day I was going to have to take the next step toward dealing with my failing kidneys. I was inching closer to major surgery.

But as divine fate would have it, I was met at the door of the kidney clinic by an associate who we'll call Lorenzo. He was the man who would do my intake and walk me through the introductory process. *Wait! I know that shirt he's wearing*, I thought. *It's last spring's Banana Republic button-down in citrine, and look at those darling little Cole Haan loafers.* His tan was hazmat orange from too many weekends at the White Party in Palm Springs. I could have sworn he was wearing the new glitter plum lip liner from M•A•C I thought: *A sister! Here! Everything is going to be just fine.*

Lorenzo knew instinctively what I needed. Like a mother hen, he immediately whisked me out of sight of the other patients. He may have only been five feet tall and barely 120 pounds but he had a fiercely protective glare and didn't hesitate to swat away anyone who looked in my direction. When we were safely alone in the elevator, he turned to me and girlishly giggled. "I know I shouldn't say this, but I know who you are, and I just *loooooooooovvvvvvvvve* you!"

It was as if I had breathed for the first time since my diagnosis. I had met an ally and confidante. Someone to lean on. After months of suffering alone, it was a gift to have met someone who was so kind and compassionate and relatable. Someone who *got* me.

"Oh thank you!" I blushed. "And I am *fainting* over the color of your shirt!"

Lorenzo brought me to Dr. Stanley Jordan's office and started to leave. *Don't leave me don't leave me don't leave me*, I was thinking. But his eyes said that it was time to cut the umbilical cord.

Dr. Jordan's cramped office was decorated in post-modern medical paper chic—towers of files, mounds of paperwork—and was devoid of any of the trappings of your average Beverly Hills physician, not even a leather club chair or a gold-framed Harvard diploma on the wall. It certainly didn't seem big enough for the head honcho of kidneys in Hollywood. (I later found out that there's a whole hierarchy of body parts at the hospital: Hearts are A-list, very Brad Pitt; and lungs are also all the rage, soooo George Clooney. But kidneys? Straight C-list. Think Carrot Top.)

As I sat there, I decided Dr. Jordan must be an ogre. After all, he would be in charge of the mutilation and destruction of my beautiful kidneys, taking away my last vestige of innocence and bringing me into the pits of surgical hell. I imagined him as a hunchback with long claws and beady little eyes, a crooked toothless slit of a mouth, knife scars across his face, maybe a hook for an arm. Worst of all, I imagined him in polyester pants with the biggest sartorial offense of all time, three pens in the pocket of his lab coat. I almost believed that he was going to rip my kidneys out then and there.

The door opened with a squeak of rusty hinges, and I jerked around and looked up to face my tormentor. And there was a dead ringer for a young Tom Brokaw standing in front of me. This man had the kindest eyes—and, even better, a flattering haircut (the number one requirement of any person who was going to be overseeing my surgery). He was wearing a lab coat—no pens!—and his pants appeared to be an acceptible lightweight all-seasons wool.

"I'm Dr. Jordan," the man said, offering his hand. As I looked in his eyes, it was the patient-doctor version of love at first sight.

Dr. Jordan was calm, warm, gracious, and immediately soothing. He looked at my kidney numbers and was extremely patient about my questions, which was a good sign. At the end of the nitty-gritty discussion, he got very real.

"This is fixable," he said, leaning forward and looking me in the eyes. "This is treatable. We have an over ninety percent success rate with our transplants."

Fixable? Fixable? You mean, not deadable? Not last-ritesable? The word bounced around my cerebellum, did cartwheels in my head. Fixable? It was like fireworks were going off. I feasted on the word fixable as though it was a medium-rare filet mignon in a lovely reduction sauce.

I'm Mr. Cynical. Usually I meet somebody and by the time they've barely said hello, I have had them Googled, fingerprinted, and followed by the FBI for a few weeks. But something special happened in Dr. Jordan's office, something extraordinary. There was an aura about Dr. Jordan that was so truthful and pure and mystical that without hesitation, I believed him.

"Howfastcanwedoit?" I blurted out, knowing that there weren't very many miles left on my kidney. I was petrified that he was going to say that it could take years.

"Things could move quickly," he said. "If you find a donor, we work fast. We want you to have the transplant as soon as possible: That's our goal. It could be a matter of months."

But first, he said, I needed to find a new kidney. Even though everyone is born with two kidneys, you only need one functioning kidney to survive, but procuring that one kidney is a formidable challenge. I was already on the national waiting list for an organ donor: Dr. Moss had put me on the list immediately after I was diagnosed. But the odds of getting a kidney soon weren't in my favor: According to the National Kidney Foundation, at any given time, roughly sixty-three thousand U.S. patients are waiting for an organ transplant. Only sixteen thousand or so transplants take place every year. Of those, roughly half of the kidneys come from cadavers: You die in a car crash and your kidneys go to people like me. But there are simply not enough of those kind of organ donors. The wait for a kidney in Los Angeles was five to seven years—and some people, tragically, had been waiting even longer for the right match. The plight of those thousands of people outraged me: Were we living in a third world country?

Because of this shortage, in recent years, doctors like Dr. Jordan had been promoting a new solution. "You should find a living donor," he told me. "Go to your friends and family and see if one of them is willing to donate a kidney to you. If you are fortunate, you can get the surgery as soon as possible." In fact, a transplant using a living donor would be more likely to be successful: Kidneys taken from cadavers had a five-year survival rate of 63 percent, while living donor kidneys survived 76 percent of the time.

"What happens when I get the new kidney?" I asked. "Will I

still be able to work? Will I be an invalid forever? Am I going to be healthy? Will my life ever go back to being normal? When can I highlight my hair?"

Dr. Jordan smiled gently. "People who have transplants can live long healthy lives. I have one patient who recently went trekking in the Himalayas."

For months, in my head, I had written the script of my kidney transplant as a horror film: Something like Bela Lugosi's classic *The Body Snatcher*, where helpless victims are killed by doctors who want to use their bodies for evil experiments. Now I was here, and where was the ugliness that I had feared? Where was the whiff of formaldehyde? Where was Bela with his bloody knife? Where was the big tank where they kept the live kidneys?

Here was reality, and the lights were still on: There were no gargoyles, no wolves roaming the corridors with bloody body parts hanging from their fangs, no ominous lightning cracking outside the window. My tragedy had faces now, and they didn't bear any resemblance to Bela or Boris Karloff. It had Dr. Jordan's empathetic face. It had Lorenzo with his little pink barrettes skipping and singing selections from *Mamma Mia* beside me.

Lorenzo next whisked me to the in-house social worker's office. She needed to make sure that I was emotionally stable enough to handle the operation, and I gave her a performance worthy of Tori Spelling in the Lifetime TV classic *Mother, May I Sleep with Danger?*

She took in the whole visage—from the gold metallic Dries man bag to my Sex Pistols *Anarchy in the UK* T-shirt—and pursed her lips. "Would you describe yourself as a stable person?" she asked. "Have you ever had mental health issues? Would people say you have a temper? On what occasions do you raise your voice? Do you own a BB gun? How do you feel about kittens? Do you like to hang out in post offices?"

"Who, me?" I replied, smiling serenely. "Stable? I just won the Zen Master of the Year prize at Gurmukh's kundalini class."

And then we had only one last ghost to wrestle with. I had to meet my surgeon, the fabled illustrious Dr. Louis J. Cohen.

I was sitting in Dr. Cohen's office nervously flipping through the latest issue of *Kidney Monthly*, absorbed in an article called "Sex Secrets of a Kidney Transplantee" when Dr. Cohen walked in the room. It was as if he came with a soundtrack of harps and singing cherubs. My surgeon—who would have my life in his hands—looked like the vision I'd always had of the Almighty. He had long white hair, like feathered angel wings. Was it central casting who sent him? It was almost like the Lord himself was here to save me.

"I'm so relieved that you don't look like an old conservative doctor," I told him. "You seem young to me, with that groovy long hair. I feel like you could come out and see some bands with me and my friends at Spaceland."

He laughed. "I'm not that young. I was a surgeon in Vietnam."

Talk about breaking the ice. "Vietnam?" I repeated.

"I was on the battlefield, performing surgeries on the spot. It was gruesome." This moved me beyond words: I imagined him on the battlefield, saving lives, and felt fortunate that my kidneys would be in his special blessed hands. He really was an experienced surgeon, to say the least. I was humbled.

The energy of the Cedars-Sinai staff was inspiring: It charged me up. For a split second, I felt as if I'd already been cured by their optimism. I left the kidney clinic that day with a sense of new resolve. *I'm not waiting anymore,* I thought, *and I'm not going to cower anymore*. I was going to get a kidney transplant as soon as possible. A warrior had come alive inside of me.

I was still in my prime, I reminded myself. I had more to do: many more dresses to lovingly critique, more blowouts to micromanage, more celebrities to accost on the red carpet. I'd never sung in front of an audience of thousands, kayaked through the rainforest, or dived out of a plane. And, of course, my number-one goal was yet to be fulfilled: I still hadn't slept with a celebrity!

It was time to get a new kidney and move on with my life. All I needed to do now was find one.

CHAPTER 4

Tyra's $10 Million Ta Tas and One Priceless Kidney

S upermodels don't get any smarter at twenty-five thousand feet above sea level. "You kind of like walk up on the runway like you're kind of fierce, but it's like a controlled fierceness," model laureate Tyra Banks expounds on the complex art of parading around in public in lingerie.

There will be no meals served today on the Victoria's Secret jet that is carrying me, Tyra, Gisele, Heidi, Adriana and Alessandra down to Miami for the next stop of the Angels in America tour, but Gisele is generously sharing her diet tonic water with me. I am the only media figure who has been annointed with an invitation to bring my camera crew on board to record this historic journey. I am here to probe the minds of the world's most famous professional poseurs, who are shilling the greatest invention since the ceramic flatiron, Victoria's Secret's new holiday gift bra.

It's November, nearly two months since my visit to the Cedars-Sinai kidney center, and I feel like I have a split personality (with only one wardrobe between them). One minute, it's Mammaries over Miami, and the next minute I'm caught up in the donor-finding process that is taking place on terra firma. Things are happening so quickly that I can barely process what's going on.

"OK, it's time for a serious question." I cozy up to Heidi Klum: "Let's talk cup sizes."

But Tyra barges in to our conversation before my little German strudel can respond, and flops a bra down in my lap. But this is not just any *brassiere*: It's the new Heavenly 70 Fantasy Bra, encrusted with 2,900 pavé-set diamonds, and with a price tag of $10 million.

"This is shaped exactly to the specifications of my body," says Tyra. "I had to get a mold done—like, had to sit there half-naked in front of a man I didn't know."

I have to put Tyra on hold because Gisele has summoned me for an audience. Gisele's brow is furrowed, as if she is pondering a serious thought, and I stop, waiting for whatever deep observation is about to fall out of her mouth. "You know," she says. "I love french fries."

I think I've had an aneurism. I want to bolt to the front of the plane, crack Tyra over the head with a seat tray, steal the diamond bra, parachute out of this plane, and go build a ten million dollar kidney center somewhere.

I dread landing in Miami, normally one of my favorite play-grounds, because I know that once I'm back on land I'm finally going to come clean to the world about my kidney disease. I can't avoid it anymore: Before I boarded the plane, I found out that I might have found a potential donor.

Finding a kidney isn't easy. You can't order one online, or have it delivered in a basket of muffins. There is only one way to get a kidney from a living donor: You have to find someone who wants to give you theirs.

The success of a kidney transplant depends on how compatible the donor and recipient are: not just blood type, but also six different antigens (which stimulate the production of antibodies and fight off disease). When we met in September, Dr. Jordan had told me that my best shot at a donated kidney would be a close family member: My parents or my sister Alisa. Not only would they be the most willing to have their own healthy kidney removed for my sake, he suggested, but they would be the most likely match.

But there was no way I was going to ask Mr. and Mrs. Cojo for a kidney, and my sister's compatibility hadn't been determined yet. My first concern was for my sweet, gentle, delicate parents. *I can't risk operating on people in their seventies,* I thought. *Under no circumstances will I put my mother and father in danger.*

All of these thoughts and anxieties haunted me through the fall, and the stress was wreaking havoc on my body. I was wired from guzzling diet soda day and night, and suffered from an insomnia that left me hypnotized by infomercials for Victoria Principal's kelp masks until dawn. I was at a standstill, unsure how to even start this whole process of announcing the news to my intimates and going begging for a kidney. I couldn't do it alone. I needed someone to support me and be my cushion as I faced the most difficult conversation I might ever have with my parents. I went back and forth and back and forth until my heart finally pulled me toward one of the safest havens I had: My best friend Abby.

Abby thinks I'm from another planet and loves me anyway. I often question whether my ultra-straightlaced friend is the secret adopted love child of Rush Limbaugh and Bill O'Reilly. On weekends she makes sandwiches for the homeless. I spend my free time getting my epidermis varnished at the dermatologist's. She knits, I cocktail. Despite being completely, totally, utterly different, Abby has always been my lighthouse, my anchor.

When I moved to Los Angeles, Abby was my first friend, the woman who knocked me into shape and taught me how to take care of myself. When I was growing up, my mother never taught me how to do household things. I was the male heir in an Eastern European family, which meant I was practically a demigod. It's such a medieval system: The daughter (i.e., my sister Alisa) is taught to cook and sew and the son (i.e., Me) isn't even allowed to tie his own tennis shoes.

This princely upbringing would come back and bite me in the derriere when I got the keys to my first Hollywood apartment. Within a week, surgical masks were required for any soul with the wherewithal to brave the delightful smells of moldy lasagna and my leaning tower of dirty socks. Abby made it through the doorway and immediately appointed herself Head of Housekeeping. She taught me what a flat sheet was. She sternly informed me that you couldn't make a suit out of steel wool. And, the worst humiliation of all, she took my toilet-cleaning virginity away from me. But she was also there for me during all the tough, rough times, when I was down and out—poor, lonely, rejected, and wearing really bad clothes.

Abby was now living in New York, where she developed television projects like Comedy Central's *Kenny vs. Spenny,* and telling her about my disease would involve bonus miles. In October, when I was in town, I invited her out to dinner at an Italian trattoria: I chose Italian, because I felt if you were going to go down you might as well do it while mainlining spaghettini puttanesca and ossobuco alla Milanese and five heaping helpings of paper-thin melt-in-your-mouth imported prosciutto—not to mention gallons of chianti. I was tempting fate by consuming alcohol, considering that my put-upon kidneys could barely process a green tea–pomegranate bran muffin anymore.

But once we were seated at the table, I couldn't face it. *Once I tell Abby, this is going to be real,* I thought, as we ate. *It won't be a bad dream anymore.* So we finished dinner without a word from me. And then I was going to tell her on the walk back home to her apartment, but I still wasn't ready. I kept putting it off. It was an unseasonably warm evening, and as we walked the quiet streets to her Upper East Side apartment, I was about to spontaneously combust from the tension. I kept telling myself, Tell her now! But then a desperate plea would echo through my brain: *No—twenty more minutes of freedom! Please! Twenty more minutes of life as I know it!*

When we arrived at her apartment I realized that I couldn't buy any more time. Her studio apartment was a maze of cardboard boxes and bubble wrap: She had only recently moved in, and there was no furniture. We sat down on orange crates and finally I blurted out: "Abby, I have some bad medical news about me. . . . I've been diagnosed with kidney disease."

Abby's breath seemed to stop. I was so struck by the look in her eyes that I couldn't even hear her response: Her entire being seemed to ache for me. She came over and put her arms around me and held me as I began to sob. For the first time in months—maybe even a lifetime—I invited the wounded creature inside of me to come outside.

Abby, always the caretaker, soon composed herself. I was still in pieces but she was already stoically contemplating a plan of attack. "What's the first step you need to take?" she asked.

"I need to have a kidney transplant," I told her. "I need to find a kidney donor."

I rattled on, explaining what the disease is and what my options were, as she listened quietly. When I was done, Abby spoke up. "*I'll give you a kidney,*" she said. "I don't even need to think twice about it."

I traveled past mere garden-variety shock and went straight into the stratosphere of amazement. I was so moved to discover that Abby was capable of so much compassion and generosity. That's what sent my circuits racing. Even if she was being a really loving friend and just saying it to comfort me, her words warmed my very being.

We went outside because we needed air and sat on the stoop of her building for a long time. We talked about all the issues—my concerns about my parents, my fears about losing my job, what a transplant would mean to my health. And sensible Abby immediately began making plans.

"We are going to take care of this," she said. And with these words suddenly I was not alone in the cage with my disease anymore. Suddenly, I was part of a "we," and that "we" was so nourishing to me: It gave me the greatest sense of relief.

I left Abby to ponder her offer. It still hadn't really hit me that she could possibly be my donor. But she never wavered from that first conversation. It was all very black and white to her, and I was relieved to heap this mountain of stress on someone. She had the clarity, and I clung to her. I still didn't know what the bigger picture would ultimately end up being: I needed to talk to my family, to consider my sibling as a donor. But, despite not knowing how it was going to end up, who was going to ultimately be giving me a kidney, we took the first steps toward finding out Abby's compatibility. Could she possibly be The One?

While Abby was undergoing the first compatibility tests in New York, I practically had a cot at Cedars-Sinai. My kidneys were failing, and my doctors were doing everything they could to sustain their life expectancy: Nearly every day I was being called into the hospital for some sort of test or shot. There were nonstop blood draws and epogen shots for anemia. I was pumped with pills to control my potassium, calcium, and blood sugar levels: When your kidneys are failing, everything in your body fails with them so every single neuron had to be inspected. The doctors were obsessed with my urine output: For one particularly gruesome test, I had to collect every drop of urine over a 24-hour period and carry it around with me in a plastic container surrounded by icepacks that I hid in my napsack. And I had made a new friend, gout.

With so many jaunts to the hospital, it was growing impossible to conceal the truth from my employers at *Entertainment Tonight*. In mid-November, I took the Kidney Confession Tour to the Paramount Lot, where I summoned my bosses—Linda Bell Blue, the executive producer; Janet Annino, then co-executive producer on *ET*; and Terry Wood, who oversees all of CBS/Paramount's domestic television. "I need to tell you something," I told Janet, "but it needs to be somewhere private."

"How private?" she asked.

"I mean *private*, think Area 51, no lip-readers in sight," I said.

It's not easy to find privacy in the offices of *Entertainment Tonight*. We looked in one conference room, and then another, but there were always people around.

"Why don't we go to New York?" I suggested.

If you've watched *Ghost* or *Seinfeld*, you've seen the New York I'm talking about: It's a perfect replica of an old New York street, permanently erected on Paramount's back lot. Lined up along the tree-shaded lane are dozens of rowhouses and musty storefronts. Look up and in the distance you'll see palm trees. It is surreal: New York City, California 90038.

I sat on the steps of a fake brownstone, in the warm fall sunshine, with Janet, Linda, and Terry, and I told them what was going on. "I don't know what I'm going to do with work; how this is going to affect my career," I said.

"No matter what happens, we're behind you," Terry assured me.

Eternally a producer, Linda immediately took charge of my transplant; "We'll get you in touch with some good doctors," she said. "We're going to make sure you get the best care."

The four of us sat there weeping. I was surprised: I'd expected anyone in their positions to see me as flawed, to say, *Take your useless kidneys and get off the lot!* Instead, surrounded by these strong, extraordinary women, I knew I was part of a unit. These powerhouses could produce anything, and they'd decided to take me on as their next blockbuster project.

As we sat there drying our eyes, a tour went by with a dozen tourists walking through the set. One woman eyed us and then ripped herself away from the group to come stand in front of us. She stared at me and then blurted out: "Are you Cojo?!"

"Yes," I replied. "Hi!"

Beside me, Linda was already on the phone with a doctor. I was still drying the tears off my face. Janet and Terry were hugging me. But the woman in front of me had more important concerns: "What do you think of my outfit?" she bubbled.

The news within *ET* began to take on a life of its own. A television interview with Mary Hart was in the works and a press release had been drafted. I had to scrounge up the courage to be so public with my illness, but I refused to spend my life in hiding: Both in my personal life, and also with my high-visibility job. Once this van was moving, there was no turning back. I was going public. It was too far gone. I wasn't going to go to Cedars-Sinai in giant sunglasses and a poly-cotton burqa forever. And it was time to tell my family, before they found out from someone else.

I'd played the scene of telling my parents in my head over and over and over again. I'd built it up to be this monumental event. I would fly them out to California. I toyed with the idea of telling them over kosher Chinese, but that seemed frivolous: I just wanted them in my living room, to somehow tell them straight on, no bells, no whistles. I imagined their arms around me and our stereophonic group weep-a-thon; they would soon break away and start praying to various deceased relatives.

But when the moment came, it wasn't the way I had planned. By the end of November, my bosses and I had concurred that it wasn't practical to contain my secret any longer, and my *ET* interview was about to air. My parents were on vacation in Israel for a month, visiting relatives. I felt nauseous as I picked up the phone to tell them. I will always feel guilty about not telling them in person, but at least, I thought, they were with family so they would have great support and comfort enveloping them.

According to Cojocaru Family Law, you don't make a call across an ocean, two seas, and a desert unless you've got a pregnancy to announce or really bad news. I could tell my mother was taken aback by the sound of my voice.

"What? What's going on?"

"Mom, I have some news," I said. My heart wasn't palpitating anymore. In the moment, I turned strong and laid out my concerns. "It's going to sound bad, but listen to me . . . everything will be OK! You have to promise me that whatever I say to you you can't start with the screaming and hysteria. I need you to be calm."

And my mother, to her infinite credit, did stay calm. "OK, I'm listening," she said.

"I went to a doctor, had some tests, and something is wrong with my kidneys," I said, slowly.

I heard a gasp on the other end of the line. "What's wrong?!" She asked.

I didn't tiptoe. "Listen, I have to have a kidney transplant," I said. "But my doctor says it's very treatable, very fixable. It's not as scary as it sounds."

I couldn't hear a sound through the phone except for her labored breathing. "Oh my God," she whispered. "Oh my God, oh my God, oh my God. This can't be. Where are you? I'm coming to you."

"No. Stay with your family. It's going to be in the news, and you are so much better off there. You'll have time to think and collect yourself."

"The news?!" she cried. "Are you crazy! Don't tell anyone! It's private!"

That I was going public seemed to send my mother over the top. It's understandable: She grew up in Holocaust Romania, where if you said the wrong word you were arrested and never seen again. You didn't air your laundry in public, not just because it wasn't polite, but also because you could end up rotting in the bottom of a pit in the woods.

"I'm not going to hide," I said. "Mother, I can't exactly go on vacation for a year, I can't pretend I'm going to Italy to study abroad. People know me."

We stayed on the phone for an hour, much of it simply not talking. I broke down. She broke down. When I hung up the phone, I was surprised by the catharsis that I felt: It hadn't been as bad as I thought. My mother may have been shocked, but I'd heard something in her voice that sounded more like strength. Now, the stage was set. I had told my parents, my friends and work, and I even had a potential donor; I was leaving Denialville and shipping my baggage to a new zip code.

When I got to the studio the day of my first public interview about my disease, the crew still had no idea why I was being interviewed. And when the interview with Mary Hart was over, everyone's jaws were hanging open. It was out there. I felt buoyed, and a little high, almost elated. I could almost see the relief oozing out of my pores. In the days that followed, a media frenzy ensued: Suddenly my kidneys were the most famous internal organs in America.

I started getting E-mails from around the world, coming from as far away as Greece, Singapore, Australia, the Philippines, and England. There were thousands of E-mails—printed out, the stack of messages was a foot tall—and I read them all. They sustained me.

From a family also with PKD, I wish you the best. I lost my mother, grandmother, and two uncles to this disease, and now one of two sisters has it. Luckily I do not; however, I know the effects and problems you must be going through. My mom had a double transplant, liver and kidney, and we lost her after forty-two days. But she was sixty-nine, and you are young, otherwise healthy, and, I believe, too full of life to let this get the best of you. Keep your head up and live every day to the fullest. You will be in my prayers.

Cojo! Wow. Last night I tuned in to ET to get my daily dose of celebrity news. When I heard about your kidney, I couldn't stop watching the show. I've had kidney disease since I was born and I was on different forms of dialysis for three years. I think it is so inspiring and brave of you to come out and let people know what kidney disease and transplants are all about. I have provided my E-mail, should you ever need a buddy to talk to.

Those E-mails were gifts that went straight to my heart. You can't imagine how it feels to know that you are the recipient of mass affection, that thousands of people with pure hearts are praying for you, lighting candles, wishing you well. I could almost feel them healing me.

I knew that going public with my disease would have some kind of impact, but only when I started receiving these E-mails did I really understand what a difference I might be able to make. When I read their letters and heard their voices in my head, I suddenly understood that I could inspire people to do something tangible about kidney disease.

Cojo, After I saw your story on ET *I was so touched by it that I filled out the donor card on my ID. May God bless you.*

I had made contact. It amazed me that just by talking about my disease, in the most simplistic of terms, I was capable of moving people into action.

In early December, a tube of Abby's blood took a flight from New York to Los Angeles and straight to Cedars-Sinai for testing. I fixated on her blood practically every minute of that week, while we waited for the test results. That week, *Entertainment Tonight* sent me to visit the "death headquarters" of Academy Award–winning makeup artist Matthew Mungle, designer of the dead bodies on *CSI*. Over the course of three hours, he made me over as a corpse in latex and fake blood. Afterward, I stared at a deathly visage of myself in the mirror and couldn't help but shiver. Abby's blood *had* to be a match.

When the call came, three days later, I was still picking latex out of my nostrils. "I have very good news, Steven," Dr. Jordan said. I could hear the smile in his voice. "Abby's a match."

"She's a match? Really?" I was laughing and crying at the same. My head was spinning so quickly I almost felt it detach and fly off my body. I hung up and called my parents.

I screamed into the phone before my mother even had a chance to say hello. "It's a match!" I screamed. "It's a match!"

I could practically hear my parents doing the cha-cha on top of the dining room table in Montreal. "I've been praying and praying! Every rabbi in Montreal has been praying!" my mother cried. I could hear her knocking on something in the background. "Touch wood, I am so happy. I love Abby!"

The next call was to Abby. "We're doing this, aren't we?" she said, when she heard my shrieking voice on the other end of the line. She didn't sound the least bit frightened.

Abby made plans to come to Los Angeles for the final tests at the end of December and if all went well, she'd move in with me until the operation in mid-January. The transplant that had always seemed so intangible was now just a matter of weeks away.

I had one final appearance on the *Today* show before the end of the year. I flew out to New York just before the holidays. It was my usual It's Cojo Time, a frothy fun segment showing the hottest products worn by celebrities: cellulite-busting jeans, J. Lo's monogrammed panties (at the time, very au courant) and Pamela Anderson's soda pop–top eco-friendly handbags.

I was giddy. I had been thrust into the limelight because of my PKD, suddenly turned into some kind of role model, and I decided that if I was going to be Kidney Boy, then I had to tell America I was alive and kicking. I had talked so seriously about PKD in all my media interviews over the previous weeks; but now I wanted to show that people with an illness could work and keep their sense of humor. I was bouncing off the walls, making over-the-top kidney jokes. I seized control of the airwaves and held an impromptu press conference. "I want everyone to know that I've named my kidneys," I announced to the nation. "Hazel and Phinneas!"

On air, I was able to let off steam, but by the time I left the studio that day, trepidation was starting to sink in. I knew that in a best case scenario, I would be bedbound for two months or more after my transplant. And even after I recovered, my life was going to be so different. As someone with a "condition," how was I going to bounce back and forth from coast to coast every week? I knew in my heart that wasn't going to work and I had to concede that there were going to be massive changes in my life. It left a sick feeling in my stomach. When I left Rockefeller Center that day, I didn't know when, or even if, I was ever going to set foot in that building again.

CHAPTER 5

Always Exfoliate Before Surgery

Abby had a prime, Grade A kidney. She was clean as a whistle. I don't think that a nun would have checked out better. She was someone who very rarely drank, never smoked, never did drugs, ate well, never stayed out late. As I told her in early January as we prepared for the transplant, "Thank you for offering your kidney, because I would have ripped that kidney out of you if you hadn't."

All of the sudden things began to move at a breakneck speed. The surgery was scheduled for January 14. My parents and my oldest friend, Shari, were coming in from Montreal. Since childhood, Shari has been my go-to person when there's a problem. Today, she's a social worker, dealing with battered and molested children, so she's dealt with the grim and the ugly. She is great in a crisis: She has the ability to really collect herself. She promised me she'd be with me every step of the way.

As excited as I was that the transplant was about to happen, I was also dreading it. I was still intact, after all, and there were even days when I could pretend I was healthy. But now I was headed into the hard part. What would that be like? They were going to cut me open! Everything that had come before this now felt like foreplay; suddenly, I knew in grisly detail about Abby's laparoscopic surgery, how many hours my transplant would take, the long, painful recovery that would happen afterward. I knew that sometimes patients received kidneys that lasted only hours before failing. Abby was saying good-bye to one of her internal organs and, now that fear was setting in, it seemed like a crapshoot. It was too much, too close.

I started to irrationally fear staying in a hospital. The only time I'd ever stayed in a real hospital was ten years before, when I moved to LA and had no medical insurance. At the time, I was chain smoking and going out and drinking; eventually I got the flu, which turned into bronchitis, which turned into pneumonia, which landed me in the downtown county hospital. At County Hospital, there were gang members coming in with gunshot wounds and police in the waiting room and blood everywhere. Delirious, I passed out, and when I woke up I was jammed in a room with twenty other male patients. We had been relegated to the Left for Dead Ward. It was dark and airless and I couldn't see the enemy. It sounded like there were wild boars all around me, snoring and flatulating and groaning in pain.

I pressed the nurse's call button frantically. No one came. In the bed next to me, a tattooed beast of a man with a head injury fixated on me with his one good eye. "Got any cigarettes?" he muttered.

"Noooo," I said in a tiny voice. "I have pneumonia."

"Bastard in that bed over there is my brother-in-law. I'm gonna kill him as soon as I can sit up."

"Ummmm . . ." I said.

I hit the nurse's call button five more times. Finally, she materialized at the foot of my bed. "I can't stay here," I whispered to her. "There are *violent* types in here. Could I get a private room?"

She thought a minute, looking at my imploring Bambi eyes, and then at the room of brutes around me. I could tell she knew I was right: I wouldn't survive the night. "There's no private rooms here," she said, taking pity on me. "But you *could* sleep in the hallway. I'll keep an eye on you."

I spent the rest of that night under the bright fluorescent lights of the County Hospital hallway, parked near the nurses station. I kept one eye cocked until the sun rose, afraid that I was going to be smothered with a pillow if I nodded off to sleep.

So this was my frame of reference: The county hospital and old movies, like *One Flew over the Cuckoo's Nest*. No wonder Mr. Melodrama was terrified. On the other hand, I had also fallen madly in love with the kidney team at Cedars. I felt so much genuine concern from them: I would walk into the clinic and their faces would light up. I would see encouragement in their eyes. If the people were so lovely, could a stay in the hospital be that bad?

And then there was Dr. Jordan, who was quickly becoming the hero of my little movie. I don't know why Dr. Jordan hadn't already put me in the psychiatric ward across the street: I don't think he'd ever experienced anything like me. When I'd initially gone to visit him, I had serious questions, the big ones like, "What is the formula for the gene code that passed this disease on to me?" and "Can I have a molecular breakdown of the cysts?" But increasingly, my questions were starting to be less of a scientific nature. It was, "Can I get a lomi lomi rub while I'm in the ICU? Transplants can be so drying on the skin," and "How soon after surgery can I have my placenta facial?"

BZZZZT! The alarm went off at three o'clock in the morning the day of my surgery, January 14. Get a Free Kidney Day had arrived. I'd woken up early to pack: Only the necessities of course. Several Juicy cashmere sweat outfits in opal and dark cocoa and winter fog gray. A Dolce & Gabbana leopard print bathrobe. Black Gucci slippers. Fake sheepskin-lined Uggs in case my toes got cold. Annick Goutal scented candles. Enough makeup to spackle the faces of an entire troupe of

America's Next Top Model aspirants. The way a seaman would pack life vests, I packed La Prairie sheer foundation.

With my surgery only a few hours away, the inside of my house was a total madhouse: My family was there, Shari was there, Abby was there. And to top it all off, Oprah's film crew waltzed in the door at 4:00 a.m. It was already clear that a lot of people were interested in hearing my story after I had my transplant. In December, I'd had an informal discussion with my *Today* show producer about doing an interview after my operation. The doctors had decided that bringing a film crew into the hospital wouldn't be safe or appropriate, and the *Today* show had sensitively agreed to wait about three weeks after my return from the hospital, in early February, to do my first live interview. I was also talking to *Entertainment Tonight* about doing a taped interview for the night before the *Today* show piece aired. And in the days just before my surgery, I had also agreed to go on Oprah's show in April, once I'd recovered, to talk about my illness. Oprah's crew had arrived to pre-tape me getting ready.

As I was packing my bathrobes, Oprah's crew was filming my every move. I'm not the type to shy away from a camera, but for once, the experience was surreal: In the rawest, most visceral moment of my life, I had a boom mike hanging a foot over my head. I was torn in two: I wanted my privacy for this intense moment, but it also was a fleeting life experience that I wanted to capture. *As long as they stay out of the operating room*, I thought: I wanted my doctors focusing on my kidneys, not worrying about whether the cameras were capturing their good side.

Still, I was holding it together. As the camera crews zoomed in on us, I turned to Shari and looked at her critically, noting the Ronald McDonald–orange lipstick she'd put on for the occasion. "That lipstick is embarrassing," I insisted. "You should have a nude lip, not an orange lip. You're blinding me, and you're going to blind Oprah."

Considering that Abby was about to undergo surgery too, she was remarkably calm and collected. She had put her life on hold for me, including her job. Her recovery from her surgery would require a four-week stay with me, and her family would be flying in to visit and take care of her. But tonight, she was the picture of Zen, as she continually looked after me and my parents, holding our hands, making sure that we felt safe.

My parents were doing what they always do: They had whipped out my mother's famous chocolate-chip cake, the pride of Romania, blue ribbon winner of the Bucharest bake-off, and were feeding Oprah's crew. My mother had brought the cake down from Montreal, wrapped in tin foil, inside a plastic bag, hidden inside a sweater in her carry on. My mother's purse is like a minibar with handles, and there is nothing—no illness, no strife, no world disaster—that can't be fixed with food. She'd come equipped with cake, bagels, and an entire brisket.

Before I got in the car to leave, I put on my lucky leather trench coat. And then we drove our little caravan down a pitch-black, deserted Sunset Boulevard toward Cedars-Sinai Hospital. I drove myself: I knew this would be the last act that I would be in full control of for a while. After this, it would be out of my soft, well-moisturized hands.

Is it any surprise that Hollywood's most glamorous hospital has a hush-hush secret entrance? I had been deemed worthy of the clandestine code, and so when I arrived, I entered the hospital via an underground passageway, used to hide the likes of Elizabeth Taylor and Julia Roberts from the prying eyes of the paparazzi. There weren't any paparazzi for me, and there wasn't a red carpet (just a concrete hallway), but it felt very Hollywood nonetheless, like having VIP tickets held at will call, or being given the password for a secret club. At the entrance, we met a representative from patient relations, a woman named Robin with black curly hair and funky eyeglasses and a warm loving energy.

I was so nervous with amped-up energy that I started blathering stupidly at the poor woman. As we took the elevator to the sixth floor, I began to babble instructions. "I'm going to need a room that's at least two thousand square feet," I told her, as we rose. "I must have indirect lighting at all times, and a double sink vanity in my bathroom, with adaptors for my hairdryer and flattening iron. Can I get a room with a baby grand and chandeliers by Baccarat?"

Robin just laughed in my face. "Nice try," she said, not unkindly "You're delusional."

I had imagined that Abby and I would have a long ritual ceremony in the lobby of Cedars: Sending her off to have her kidney removed was a big deal and I had envisioned a tearful farewell. But once we got upstairs, Abby was whisked off so fast that I didn't even get a chance to say good-bye properly. She had to be prepped and then undergo her surgery before they would start on me, so that the kidney was fresh and piping hot when I was ready for it. I didn't have a room ready yet. Instead, Shari, my parents, and I waited in Robin's office while she took Abby up to the operating room.

Robin's office was very cramped. There was really nothing in it: A small windowless cube of a room, blank walls, a desk, a computer, and a few chairs. The four of us sat there, staring at each other, growing increasingly nervous. When I looked at my parents, all I saw was four eyeballs boring into me.

My parents and I had struck a bargain in advance: "I want chipper! Happy! Sunny! Think Prozac!" I'd instructed them. "I don't want you to be *real*: I want you to be uplifting! Behind my back you can have broken hearts, but I can't handle it in person." They'd understood the pact—and to their credit, have mostly upheld it to this day—but in that moment, they looked like wounded birds, and just looking at them was giving me a lump in my throat. Their ashen faces were drained of all color, their watery eyes were holding back tears, and I could feel their pain along with them. I was scared, and looking at them made it worse.

In order to calm them down, I kept repeating comforting platitudes. "It's going to be OK," I told them. "It's going to be fine. The doctor said I'm young and strong, and this doctor is not lying. It's not a big deal." But inside I was saying to myself, This is a *very* big deal. What if something goes wrong with Abby, or with me?

Thankfully I had Shari. She knew exactly what I needed at that moment. Shari and I have this unbelievable ability—despite all of our responsibilities, our families, our careers—to revert to being tittering fifteen-year-olds in the blink of an eye. We could have dealt with the moment with gravitas and dignity; instead, we turned into juveniles. We surfed the Web in Robin's office, visiting the online homes of Louis Vuitton and Chanel and Bottega Veneta. We went to the virtual makeup counter at Barneys New York and I redid Shari's face completely. We decided in the hour before my transplant that she was more of a spring than a winter. We were giddy with adrenaline and anxiety; our nervousness was taking us to the verge of hysteria.

At one point, Shari turned and looked at me critically. "Do you realize you are still wearing a full face of makeup?" Oprah's camera crew was gone, but I still looked like a painted diva from *La Traviata*. "You need to go to the washroom and scrub that all off before you go in to surgery!" she commanded. I objected. Why not look my best for the doctors, too? But she was right. I didn't want to risk any kind of infection.

By the time Robin returned to retrieve me, Shari and I were laughing uncontrollably: Being infantile had taken the edge off and calmed me down, although my parents, still terrified, weren't at all amused. But the moment had arrived. "We have to get you prepped," Robin said, soberly. Before she had even finished speaking, the four of us were on our feet, ready to go: After three hours of waiting, we just wanted to get on with it.

My private pre-op suite wasn't exactly private or a suite: it was more like a minimum security prison, with four other patients sharing the room with me, each of us waiting for our moment under the knife. I was given a bed, a bag for my possessions, and a hospital gown. When I'd thought of the hospital gown, I'd imagined something classy—maybe something in a tasteful shade of ecru, a discreet Cedars-Sinai monogram over the heart. What I got was a cheap paper tablecloth from the Beef Barn. "One size fits all" was hardly a bespoke suit: I was showing more skin than Tara Reid dancing on top of a bar at a *Girls Gone Wild* reunion in Rosarita Beach.

I lay down on the gurney they'd prepped for me, and that's when it hit me that I was about to have a *kidney transplant*. The words kidney transplant are so big that it's hard to process them. I began saying it in my head, and then saying it out loud. *Kidney transplant!* "Kidney transplant!"

I'd brought a small book of prayers with me. At this moment, being spiritual felt very necessary, and I'd requested that one of the hospital's rabbis come up to talk to me. But he turned out to be a Jungian rabbi. All I wanted was the basic menu: the prayer, the comfort, and done. Instead, when I asked him to pray for me he turned around and lashed into me: "You need to let go of the self and pray for good health for the world," he said. "There should be no 'me' involved."

"Excuse me, Deepak Chopra-with-a-yarmulke," I said, incredulously. "I'm surprised you're not selling me enlightenment CDs and meditation candles."

He walked away in a huff, probably on his way to bar mitzvah Madonna's son Rocco.

I was traumatized instead of comforted by him, but I got the solace from my parents. They had come in the pre-op room, where the three of us prayed together. It was practically a revival. We sat there, in the chilly room, hidden by the curtain that separated the hospital beds, and held hands. Anyone listening in would have heard a cacophony of singing, humming, and chants in a mix of Romanian, Hebrew, English, a nice helping of Yiddish, and I think I might have thrown in a French designer's name or two.

Praying seemed to calm my parents. In the final moments before the surgery, there were no hystrionics, no weeping at my feet. As scared as I was, I was starting to feel safe. It was beautiful to be with my family. There was so much love that it gave me peace.

By this time, the drugs they'd given me were starting to kick in. I felt dreamy and giggly. *This isn't so bad*, I thought, as the nurses arrived to wheel me in to the operating room.

When I'd imagined the operating room, I'd hoped for something from *Grey's Anatomy*: moody, atmospheric, like a good table on the patio of the Ivy on a late June evening. Incredibly gorgeous trainee doctors with perfect hair and luminous skin, huddled around, examining my charts. But this was heavy duty. It was so white and so clinical. There were at least a dozen people in the room, mostly strangers, clanking around, busy little bees with their gleaming scalpels and enormous machines. I looked at the equipment, drinking it all in. Thanks to the drugs, everything was hyperrealized and hypermagnified: the lights seemed ten times brighter, it was as cold as the polar ice caps. And the room was as noisy as the floor of a cruise ship casino, with everything beeping and clanging and ringing. But, surprisingly, the mood in the room was calm: light, rather than intense or heavy. The doctors and nurses were just there to do their job, and I found, in this last moment, that I completely trusted them.

As I lay there, growing foggier by the minute, I said my prayers and good-byes in my head. It wasn't in my hands any longer. I didn't know what shape I'd wake up in—maybe the surgery wouldn't work, and they would cryogenically freeze me instead, and I'd wake up in five thousand years—but as I lay there, I finally felt serene. There had been a knot in my stomach for so long as I tried to stay calm and cool and crack jokes for everyone, even while I was a mess inside. I had fought the fight, helped my family, dealt with my professional issues, been prodded, poked, and had my weight in blood taken, and now I didn't have to do any more work. The type A, tightly wound, anal retentive, micromanaging alpha male with control issues had nothing left to do but let go.

I have no memory of the surgery at all, though I was told it took five hours and was deemed a complete success.

I also have no memory of being wheeled in to the recovery room, where I was put next to Abby, and we held hands, and I thanked her for the beautiful gift of life she'd given me. "I'm alive," I apparently said to her. "Are you alive?"

And I have no memory at all of waking up for the first time in my hospital room, with my friends and family around me. In fact, the first clear post-operation memory I have is of the following morning, when I awoke, looked down to see the incision at the base of my stomach, and discovered that I'd had my very first Brazilian bikini wax courtesy of Cedars-Sinai's ace surgical team. I was Steven Cojocaru from the neck up, and Dakota Fanning from the waist down.

CHAPTER 6

Dude, Where's My Catheter?

'd had a pep talk with myself before I went into the hospital. I was
not going to raise my usual ridiculous, royal demands. I promised myself, no checking the thread count on the hospital sheets;
nary a complaint about the channel selection on the television or
the sandpaper towels; not a squeak about not being able to ring up
for French onion soup and a banana-espresso milkshake at two in
the morning.

But mere hours after my epic surgery, all these vows vanished.
Eyes at half-mast, speaking in morphinized tongues, I was wheeled
into my hospital room. I don't remember much, but Shari later told
me that my gravelly, drug-addled voice immediately boomed out
from the bed: "This room is *disgusting*."

In regressive therapy, I can call it up now: My room was the size
of a voting booth, and meat-locker cold. It was painted a ravishing
new color of mucus that's not yet in Ralph Lauren's color palette for
DuPont. The sliver of a grimy window offered a view straight into
a construction site, where jackhammers were pounding. Just on the
other side of the wall, steel girders were being pummelled together.

Barely coherent, I buzzed for the nurse.

"Yes?" she said, over the intercom.

"I need to change my room," I apparently told her. "This room is
not acceptible. I'm moving within the hour. And oh, bring me some
Vicodin on ice."

If healing is a spiritual process, I thought, then how could I possibly heal here? Maybe it was the drugs, but I had a sick obsession with my accommodations, maybe because I knew the best kept secret in town: That Cedars-Sinai has its very own enclave, a pied à terre for VIPs—the fabled and hush-hush Club Floor.

There, the rooms aren't just rooms, they are suites worthy of the Four Seasons, with million-dollar panoramic views of Hollywood. On the Club Floor, you get polished wood floors, cozy couches for lounging, and a dining room table should you want to read the trades in your bathrobe while feasting on eggs Benedict with hollandaise. Best of all are the boudoirs with lighted mirrors, with more megawattage than Jessica Simpson's bicuspids.

A C-section will get you to the Club Floor, if you're a VIP. So will cholera, a flesh-eating virus, or a wandering spleen. A kidney transplant, however, will not get you there: All transplant patients—whether they have lost a kidney or a lung or a heart—are ensconced on the Transplant Floor, where the transplant specialists are.

Certainly, I was extremely grateful to be alive, and to be on any floor, bottom line. But shamefully, as much as I tried to suppress and hide the diva in me, I sickly, inappropriately, got competitive. If Gwen Stefani's uterus was on the Club Floor, why couldn't my kidney? Why was I in steerage, stuck with the graham crackers?

Abby's kidney had taken to my body immediately. Hearing this, the night after my transplant, I experienced a pure shot of joy—I had a new kidney in me! I had arrived at the other side of this illness: I felt like I had sailed across the treacherous Pacific in a canoe and managed to land safely on the beaches of Hawaii in time for happy hour. But I didn't have time to break out the champagne and the kidney shaped ice cream cake from Baskin-Robbins. There was work to be done: I had to heal.

Lying there in the hospital bed, the reality of my situation hit me. I was hooked up to a half-dozen machines—an EKG monitored my heart, and a blood pressure monitor squeezed my arm every fifteen minutes, keeping me from getting in a good nap. I had an IV, an oxygen tube in my finger, and a catheter jammed into my John Steinberg. A constant stream of nurses and doctors trudged in and out, jotting notes, staring at machines, taking down numbers. They all wore face masks—my immune system had been compromised by the kidney transplant and they didn't want any germs to endanger the vulnerable new kidney—which made me realize how precarious my situation really was.

And I was in excruciating pain. I could barely sit up: I felt like I had been run over by a Yukon. I was bandaged, so I couldn't see the incision that stretched across my abdomen, but even through the fog of painkillers I could feel the stabbing pain. I couldn't even adjust myself to get more comfortable: Any body movement at all was unbearable.

My first night in the hospital, I was too terrified to be alone: I insisted that the nurse roll cots into my room so that Shari and my mother could stay with me, and my father slept in the waiting room just outside. Something had shifted, both physically and emotionally, when I was on that operating table, and I was still terrified by what I had become. I left the surgery with a new identity: I was now a patient, a transplantee. I had joined a new club.

The second Abby was allowed to get out of bed, the day after the surgery, she came to visit me. The nurse brought her in a wheelchair. It struck me that Abby looked like a woman who had just given birth: She had a glow to her. Her eyes were lit up and sparkling. I had never seen her smile like that, a beautiful, peaceful, happy, fulfilled smile. Even though she was in pain, her spirits were very high. And within minutes, we were cracking jokes and giggling, defusing our pain with humor.

My nurse, Dorina, told me what was up. She was a no-nonsense kind of lady. "We need to get you walking," she said, when she came in to see me on Friday night. "We have to wake up your organs, because they've been sleeping for a very long time. Walking is one of the keys to recovery."

On Saturday morning, Dorina hooked up my portable IV, and Shari and I went for our first walk. I realized, quickly, how we take things for granted—things like walking, or going to the bathroom. Suddenly, I could do neither.

"Concentrate on your breathing," Shari told me, as we inched down the hall. "It will distract you from the pain." Trust me: When you are in that much pain, nothing can distract you, but I didn't stop, and I didn't rest in chairs along the way. I was proud of myself for sticking with it.

My commitment to my recovery was one thing, but living with a catheter was another: I wanted that thing out of my body. "It's robbing me of my manhood!" I complained to Dorina. "I might never be able to use my penis again. What if it leaves me with a deformed, lopsided peter? What if I get an erection and the catheter pops out and into a nurse's eye?" Dorina, however, would have none of it: My urine was one of the best ways that they had to measure how fast I was recovering, and nurses arrived several times a day to examine its color and quantity. A full bucket was cause for celebration: It meant my kidneys were functioning. So instead I made it my goal to have the nicest urine of anyone on the floor: It had to be yellow, with a hint of marigold.

To amuse ourselves, Shari and I had come up with nicknames for everyone on the staff. There was the Troll, a squat little nurse who harassed me constantly about what I wanted to eat for lunch. The nurse with the untamed mess of fried, bleached-blonde platinum hair and bleeding red lipstick was immediately dubbed Courtney Love. The male nurse with the Russian accent and the piercing blue eyes was Mikhail Baryshnikov. The only people who escaped our nicknames were Dr. Jordan, and Jenny, my kidney coordinator: They were exempt, because they were perfect. They loved their resident diva, and I did everything I could to entertain them (and myself).

Grimly wiling the hours away, I looked at them for distraction and validation. They would come in and ooh and aah, proudly, that the color was coming back into my face. What they didn't know was that their little medical minx got up just a few minutes early on those days—maybe, around 3:45 a.m.-ish—and put on just a touch of brightening makeup . . . just a smidge, really. Just some sheer fluid foundation. Plus a little Stephane Marais concealer. A little bit of Dermalogica eye cream, Chanel mascara in Noir, Nars blush in Orgasm. Some M•A•C hush luminizer painted on top of my cheekbones, with a touch of Clarins bronzer. On my eyes? Just a drop of color: Anastasia eyebrow pencil, eyebrow brush, and world-famous eyebrow gel. Oh, and three different eyeshadows: a rainbow courtesy of Dior, Lorac, and Laura Mercier. A dusting of powder by Bobbi Brown. Face primer by Shiseido. Fake mink eyelashes by Shu Uemura. And finally, topping it all off: nostril shine diminisher by Pinkie Swear.

I might not have bothered going to all the effort, because other than the nurses and the kidney team, no one else was allowed to visit me: My doctors were concerned about the germs visitors might carry in from the outside world, and I was basically quarantined. Only my family was coming to visit; even Abby was gone, having been released from the hospital after only two days. I had visions of bringing the party to me—maybe grilling up some baby back ribs and wieners in my hospital room, hosting a potato sack race and an open bar, but that was not to happen. I wasn't even allowed flowers in my room. Instead, my room became Willie Wonka's chocolate factory: It seemed like half of Brentwood had sent chocolate macaroons, chocolate bagels, chocolate menorahs. Other people sent balloons, so many balloons that we began to fear that we would asphyxiate from them. (I donated them all to the children's ward downstairs, where they would be better appreciated.)

I was hungry for human contact, but part of me was happy that no one could come visit: I didn't want people to see me as less than I was, so vulnerable and sick. Despite putting forth my best face for the staff, the truth was that I was emotionally drained and ached all over. Thank God for the most beautiful thing in the world: the morphine drip. I was pushing that button way before my next allotment. Ten seconds after I got one dose, I would push it again to no avail. And again. And again. I wanted to be numb: I wanted a holiday from emotional pain, I wanted to feel light and floaty. In my opinion, there is no nobility in pain; there's nothing heroic about saying I'll live with it and suffer. No, I'm too much of a wuss for that. I'd take a morphine drip for a papercut if I could.

The walks grew a little easier—feeling better, I'd swapped out my bathrobe for the cashmere sweatsuit—but they were always desperate, dark moments. When I ventured out to walk I couldn't avoid the other patients. I was surrounded by ailing patients waiting for liver and lung transplants, patients whose lives were draining away from them. I could see it in their skin and in their eyes, and it haunted me. I could hear the lung cancer patients hacking nonstop. I didn't want to look: I didn't want to see it. I was just beginning to cope with my illness, and I couldn't handle anyone else's. I had to get home.

The third night of my stay at Cedars-Sinai, Shari and I "attended" the Golden Globes. Shari had seen how visibly devastated I was not to be on that red carpet, and she gleefully suggested that we have our own Golden Globes party right there in room 603C. I felt like a child invited to a birthday party with ponies, a carousel ride, and pink cotton candy. One special privilege at Cedars-Sinai—regardless of what floor you're on—is the "deluxe menu." This is a glamorous a la carte meal, as decadent as anything that you might be served at a chic restaurant in the Left Bank of Paris. Tonight was the night, we decided, to splurge: With my doctor's permission, we ordered filet mignon and potato souffle. For dessert we had, hands-down, the world's richest chocolate cake. I knew I was eating better than the attendees of the Golden Globes with their rubber banquet chicken. Shari took the edge off with a bouqueted glass of crisp French sauvignon blanc. I relished my sparkling apple cider; in my mind, I was swilling Louis Roederer Cristal 1990 Krug.

Our meal was rolled in on a special cart, decorated with a tablecloth and freshly cut calla lilies. "It's Versailles a la carte!" I beamed. As we tore into the freshly baked baguette, and watched the actresses swan by in their dresses on the television set, we could pretend we were on the red carpet with them. Lucky Shari got a blow-by-blow critique of the gowns floating by—her own personal Cojo's Top Five Best and Worst. As much as it hurt to raise my hand with an IV needle jabbed into my forearm, I applauded Uma in her light-as-air white goddess gown and screamed out, "Celestial! Quelle

Grandeur!" I got a muscle spasm in my neck when Nicole Kidman desecrated the red carpet in a one-shouldered *feathered* monstrosity. "Someone feed some bread crumbs to that runaway cockatoo!" I bellowed.

On Tuesday morning, after five nights in the hospital, I was released. Dr. Jordan came by first, checked my vital signs, and bade me farewell. "Jenny is going to come by before you leave," he told me. "She needs to teach you how to take your drugs."

This is something I hadn't considered before. In the hospital, they had been constantly giving me drugs, but I had no idea what they were. *How hard can it be?* I thought. *I've been known to take codeine to soothe the anguish of a bad, patchy spray tan.* When Jenny arrived in my room early that afternoon, she had a bag of pills with her that was the size of a Goyard weekend bag. I shut off *One Life to Live* and yawned as she sat down next to me. My brain was already preparing the celebratory bath I planned to take when I got home.

"These are your drugs," Jenny said. "And you are going to have to start taking them, on your own. It's a whole progam, and you have to be prepared, it's a lot of work. I'm here to take you through it."

Antirejection pills, she explained, are immunosuppressive drugs designed to affect your immune system so that it doesn't reject a new kidney, specifically, by suppressing your white blood cells. And then she showed me the list: Pages of handwriting, covered with lines and graphs and columns, lists of times and dosages, names of pills. First, I was to get up and take two antirejection pills on an empty stomach. I had to wait half an hour for them to get into my blood stream. Then I had to hurry and shovel down breakfast, and then, on a full stomach, take the secondary pills. By midmorning, I would be gobbling handfuls of pills: two kinds of blood pressure medication, cholesterol medication, calcium pills, pills for gout. There were enormous quantities of steroids. There were certain pills that had to be taken before lunch, and then more, immediately after lunch. Late in the afternoon I was to take two different kinds of syrup. And then the whole process would happen again at dinnertime.

I was about to tinkle in my pants. No matter how much the doctors had warned me about the lifelong commitment to antirejection pills, I had thought it would be no big deal: a couple pills washed down with tequila before I headed out to the clubs. But the chart she gave me looked like the seating chart of the *Vanity Fair* post-Oscars party. As I looked at it, it just became one big blur, and I started to get a sick feeling in my stomach. My head started spinning. *It's too much, I can't memorize* it, I thought.

This was going to be my life? This was horrific. It was a full-time job. I would need to go to pharmaceutical college to understand it.

"It's important that you are compliant," Jenny emphasized. "There's no margin for error. You cannot miss your antirejection pills." Compliant is a big buzzword in the kidney world. There are lots of patients who do not take their drugs, do everything wrong, don't exercise, and lose their kidneys as a result. The doctors don't want to waste their time and valuable resources on uncooperative and irresponsible patients.

When Jenny left, Shari and I just looked at each other. "How am I going to do this?" I said. "The only thing I can think, Shari, is that you are going to have to leave your family for a couple years, and your job, your tenure, and move to LA to be my personal pharmacist."

When I left Cedars-Sinai that morning, I had mixed emotions. I was excited that I was going home. I kept reminding myself that I was a walking miracle. But there were a lot of question marks floating around my head, a lot of fear coursing through my veins: What was in store for me? What was going to happen with my life? Was I going to be a pill-dependent prisoner to this disease?

The nurse wheeled me out to my parents' car in a wheelchair, as I clutched the enormous bag of pills. I slid into the backseat and lay down.

"We're going home!" my mom beamed. "I'm so excited. Aren't you excited, darling?"

With my friend Linda following in her car, and more friends and relatives trailing behind, it was a motorcade worthy of the Maharaja of Bengali. With a clanging bell in one hand and a bullhorn in the other, my mother had no problem sending pedestrians scurrying: "Precious cargo coming through!" A woman in a van refused to clear the way for our car, and my mother popped her head out of the sun-roof and screamed: "Move out of the way! Did *your* famous son just have a kidney transplant!?"

My mother's chirping enthusiasm filled up the empty space that my silence left in the car. The bag of pills was heavy in my lap. I looked at it and sighed. I closed my eyes and imagined throwing the pills out the car window, one by one, as we drove toward home. I could almost see the pharmaceutical trail I would leave behind, and the delicious sight of those dreaded capsules being flattened by a Proactiv-using punk in a banana-yellow Hummer, as he rolled obliviously down the Hollywood streets.

CHAPTER 7

Coping with Concealer

I may have been released from Cedars-Sinai, but I was moving directly to another hospital: Cojocaru Clinic, a maximum-security facility with two elderly Jews on guard and a moat made of chocolate-chip cake. I had two months—minimum—of quarantined recovery at home before I could even contemplate going back out into the world again. I still could hardly walk, I couldn't lift anything more than a toothbrush, and I could barely sit up. Because I was still susceptible to germs, my house had been sanitized. I was allowed only limited outside visitors, and the only times I could leave home were for my hospital checkups. Even then, I had to wear a hospital mask.

Taking care of me would be an all-consuming, brutal, twenty-four-hour-a-day job: I needed someone to clean my wound, take me to the restroom, help me get dressed, and bathe me. (Abby, who would be recovering in my guest room, was in similar shape.) There was no one else in the world I trusted to care for me more than my parents. I was incredibly fortunate that Mr. and Mrs. Cojo had willingly dropped their lives in Montreal and were moving in for the next few months to nurse me.

I desperately needed my parents: Weak and near-lifeless, I clung to them, and they were ready to give everything they had to me. But underneath, I was torn. I hadn't lived under the same roof as my parents since I fled into the night after college in order to save my sanity; and I still had disturbingly vivid flashbacks (and the occasional nightmare) about how my gigantic, artistic spirit—not to mention hair—hadn't fit into the confines of their small, all-enveloping household.

According to my parents and their Bible, *Dr. Spock's Guide to Completely Smothering and Castrating Your Son*, having your children as physically close as possible reduces risks of heart attacks and certain cancers. Growing up, the word *privacy* was not in my parents' vocabulary, and they would do anything—including telling white lies—to keep their son in close proximity.

When I was eight years old, my parents moved my family to a new house. "Oh, Steven, wait until you see our new house!" Mrs. Cojo gushed. "You're going to have your *own bedroom*."

"But all my friends are in this area," I said. At eight, I couldn't imagine anything worse than being ripped away from my neighborhood and rescinding my title of Most Hotly Sought Out Playdate of Bedford Street.

My mother realized this was going to be harder than she thought and went into full time-share salesman mode. And the bribery began. "Darling! Oy, you're going to have a room so big it's practically it's own wing! It's just like the Waldorf-Astoria, where we stayed last Passover, remember?"

"How big did you say? Tell me in square feet."

"Biiiig! You could practically put a skating rink in it," she laughed. "Oh! And you should see the bay windows!"

Hmmmm. I perked up. She had my attention. "Throw in a television and a Beta machine and it's a deal," I said.

The day that we moved in, I galloped up the stairs, frothing at the mouth, I was so eager to see my very own bedroom, my new

Shangri-la. I flung the door open and stopped cold. Surely, this must be the linen closet? My head spun around as I took it in—all three hundred square feet of it, highlighted by a crack of a window that looked out to a brick wall. A bed was pushed up against the tissue-thin wall, and directly on the other side of the wall was my parents' bed, so close that we could almost share an electric blanket. To call that room my own bedroom was laughable: Really it was an alcove attached to my parents' bedroom with a door thrown in as an after-thought.

I was still hoping that this wasn't really my room, but I looked down, and there was a box spilling over with my personal posses-sions: my custom-made tutu and my pogo stick, my Fisher-Price toy oven, and my Batman and Robin underoos.

"MAAAAAAAA!" I screamed. "We've got a problem!"

In the years that followed, being able to hear my father clip his toenails and my mother's full-blast allergy attacks in the middle of the night grew a little too cozy for me. It really became problem-atic when I hit puberty: Tissue-thin walls don't lend themselves to choking the kosher chicken. I had to come up with a new silent masturbation technique, a strict discipline with absolutely no body movement, no heavy breathing, and no bedspring squeaks: Sting would later call this tantric love, but he and Trudi never had to worry about his mother breaking down the door brandishing an inhaler, screeching "I heard a noise!? Are you having an asthma attack?"

Despite her cameo appearances in my petit boudoir—maybe even because of it—my mother and I had an otherworldly bond. I adored her delicious, colorful, no-holds-barred personality. But our overwhelming love also led to flared tempers and epic battles of will. Our fights were nothing short of operatic.

Now, all these years later, the fear of that claustrophobic love still haunted me. I was so fortunate that the people voted Greatest Parents of the Year seventeen years and running by the Romanian edition of *Parenting* magazine had dropped their lives to come utterly devote themselves to me. But I couldn't help but ask myself if I could cope with this as a grown man. What had happened when I was a kid was an issue forever stuck in my psyche: My therapist calls it the Paper-Thin-Wall-Jailed-Child-Diva Syndrome. And this time, I couldn't fall back on my teenage shenanigans of screaming, running out, and slamming the door: Instead, I was bedbound, helpless, and unable to escape. I had to confront my issues with my family dead on.

My long-suffering mother was thrilled to play the role of nurse-maid, and we quickly fell into a routine. In the morning, my father would bring his famous French toast a La Benny in to me on a tray. My father is quite the gourmet: a great cook and genius at presentation. In another life he would have been Emeril. At my house, every morning was like room service at the Ritz-Carlton. There were lovely linen napkins with napkin holders, fine china, and the morning paper neatly folded next to my breakfast on the tray.

After breakfast, my mother would start nudging me: "We have to go for a walk!" I would avoid it as much as possible: I was weak and I wanted to stay in that bed, the safest place I knew. But she would keep coming back, standing patiently by my bed in her adorable pink and fuschia hooded sweat suit from Target.

I would turn into a child and whine. "I don't have strength. I can't breathe."

And she would say, "Come on, honey. Come on. You have to!"

Only my mother could have gotten me through those walks. It was astonishing how delicate and fragile I was. Just getting ready to go for the walk felt like running a marathon. Putting on sweatpants was *work*. And then there was climbing the stairs to the front door: I had bought my three story Spanish style house in the Hills as a last-ditch effort to get my rear in shape: I figured running up and down stairs all day long would give me the high, rock hard glutes I'd always dreamed of. It didn't work. Instead, it just complicated my recovery. Every day, I had to climb those stairs, in order to build my stamina. That's how I measured my progress, if I could walk up a flight.

At first, I could only go thirty feet before I was completely sapped. My walks with my mother consisted of walking out the front door, barely making it to my next-door neighbor's, and turning back. The pain was so excruciating, throbbing and constant, that I couldn't fathom going any farther. But my mother had been drilled by the doctors about how vital it was that I walked: The more you're in bed, the sicker you get; the more you get out of bed, the faster you recover. As much as I wanted to, I couldn't be the self-indulgent invalid lounging in bed all day. She pushed me, and I begrudgingly listened.

Physically, the walks were healing me; but it was the emotional awakening that was most unexpected. This time with my mother grew sacred. My walls came down and my defensiveness ebbed away. After a lifetime, we were finally talking as adults, a new kind of communication with a different kind of tenor. We talked about where our hearts were, and how in our darkest times, when we didn't know who what when where or why, we both had incredible faith in something bigger than us, something divine.

It was on these walks that my mother really opened up to me for what felt like the first time: About what her disappointments in life were, the things she'd never wanted to burden her children with. She told me stories about being a child of the Holocaust, and being spit on by other schoolchildren for being a Jew; she talked about her father being sent off to a labor camp while her mother, with two little girls, lived on a diet of bread, water, and fear. She spoke of the challenges of being immigrants in a strange country, and surviving by spending late nights hunched over a sewing machine making dresses for rich women. We talked about survival and we patted each other on the back for making it through this crisis, better than we both thought. This situation gave us valuable time that maybe we never would have had otherwise.

My recovery was literally measured step by step. At the beginning of our walks, I huffed and puffed after reaching the next house over; then it was five houses; then the benchmark was ten, and so on. Before the surgery, I was always in such an endless hurry that I never noticed my neighbors. But as my mother and I became fixtures on the street, I began to see my neighborhood with different eyes. All the neighbors would ask how I was feeling, and I felt a kindness, almost like we were being cheered on to the finish line. I had found my Mayberry in the middle of Hollywood, and I rather liked it.

After our walk, I would collapse into my bed. Chef Mr. Cojo would gleefully deliver lunch to me, before I'd even finished digesting breakfast. I'd spend the afternoon in bed, in a painkiller daze, watching soap operas and using my special gift of X-ray Plastic Surgery Vision to while away the time: I could tell exactly how many cc's of Botox were in each actress's forehead, how much Restylane was in their nasolabial folds, and who had a newly bobbed nose (or in Hollywood propagandese, a "deviated septum repair"). The only contact I had with the ouside world came twice a week, when I put on my surgical mask and left the house to see the doctor for blood tests and a checkup.

Otherwise, I spent my afternoons on the telephone. I would call

Shari, who had returned to Canada, with updates about the Big Shave. "How is the comeback going?" she would crack. "Major growth today," I'd reply. "I guess there was sunshine." Or "Bad crop this week."

Late afternoon was Abby time for me. Abby was sequestered in the other bedroom, going through her own pain. I hadn't anticipated this. Abby has always been so self-sufficient, constantly cleaning and cooking for everyone else. Now, she was stuck in bed, in a lot of agony, and it was hard for me to see her like this; yet, her spirit was really positive and she rarely complained. I would crawl into her room, cuddle up in her bed, and we would watch television together. It was our version of cocktail hour. I couldn't stop thanking her for the gift she had given me: I would offer to wash her car for life, give on-the-spot pedicures, shoulder rubs, any purse she wanted. But she kept saying, every day, "All I want is for you to be well."

The big event of the day was dinner. My parents would spend all day making it, until the smell of beef bouillon permeated the house. My parents were champion choppers: The chopping began in the morning and went on all day. I believe it was the outlet for their fear and anxiety: Chopping, chopping, chopping, whether bell peppers or onions or tomatoes. It reverberated off the walls and interrupted my naps. Mad, loud dicing and slicing.

I looked forward all day to those candlit feasts with Abby and my parents. Those dinners were a beacon of light, the highlight of my day. I would put on a fresh hoodie, brush my hair, spritz some Creed behind my ears. I was going out. This was my night on the town.

At the end of the night, after their two-hour dinner clean-up, my mom would come down to my bedroom to change bandages and clean my surgery wound, and then help me get ready for bed. She was relentless: "Brush your teeth! Take your meds!" She waited patiently while I took care of my lengthy nighttime beauty routine—slathering on moisturizer and various other age-combating lotions. And then we would watch *Sex and the City* reruns while she rubbed my feet to take away the pain. Carrie Bradshaw was very healing. It was one giant leap for our relationship: We'd really come a long way that we could sit there together watching Samantha offering fellatio techniques to Charlotte and Miranda and not bat an eyelash.

Next door, my father would be calling—"Come to bed already! You've had a long day!"—but she would just sit there, massaging my toes and chatting with me. And for everything I did, for all the pushing and fighting to get somewhere in my career, for all the moxie and confidence and being fearless enough to move to a country and city where I knew no one—for all that, when I was in such a vulnerable state, I reverted to being a child again. And I liked it.

But those were in the good moments. And then, there were the steroid moments.

Two weeks into my recovery, I was getting better: I was still extremely weak, but I was more lucid. But then the steroids kicked in. No one had warned me about what happens when you are taking 60 mg of prednisone a day—a staggeringly high quantity—a drug that is often used by transplant patients because it reduces inflammation of the organ and helps prevent rejection. I was on a major drug trip. One side effect of taking that many steroids was that I was starting to gain weight. I was retaining so much water that my stomach was bloated and distended; another was that I had become a crazy person, ping-ponging from moments of euphoria to nervousness to depression to intense, overwhelming anger.

I became the king of the temper tantrum: the slightest things could

set me off. My parents were at the receiving end of most of my irrational mood swings: In my steroid fog, somehow it was the most
therapeutic, cathartic thing in the world to blame everything on them.
Even the most minor irritations could trigger my screaming fits: My
mother flinging the bedroom door open *without knocking* in order
to deliver laundry while I was on the edge of my bed waiting for a
major climax on my soap (were Jessica and her split personality, Tess,
going to agree on a lipstick shade?); my father interrupting my nap
with the third turkey-pastrami sandwich snack of the day. If the maga-
zines weren't stacked in alphabetical order—if *Vogue* was placed before
Harper's Bazaar—my veins would bulge with fury.

Then came moments when I was really hyper. The drugs gave
me so much energy I would push myself too hard. I would walk too
fast and come home with my kidney area throbbing and worry: *I
just damaged my kidney.* (During those first few months, that worry
eats you alive. Any wrong move, and you convince yourself you've
damaged the kidney.) I would be hot, my heart would be palpitating, and I couldn't catch my breath. I was so uncomfortable that I
wanted to rip my skin off, scratch myself, pull my hair out.

And other days, I would sink into the lows and that's when I had
to start taking tranquilizers: Valium, Xanax, not to mention Percocet and Vicodin, which I was popping for the pain. Some people
hate pills—but I *loooooved* them. The good ones, like the painkillers
and the barbiturates, were my friends. I liked the buzz: Taking pills
numbed me. They kept me calm and helped me sleep, even if they
only temporarily took the edge off of my wild emotions.

In early February, three weeks after my kidney transplant, the *Today*
show called to ask me to go on the show and talk about my recovery.

I should have known better than to try to manage my own television comeback when I barely had my mental faculties and was still crushing Demerol into my cereal. But it didn't matter anyway, because two days later, they let me go. I was blindsided. On the list of Top 5 Worst Days of My Life, this was near the top.

Before I went in to surgery, I'd told the *Today* show that I would go on air after the operation to talk about my recovery. There was a handshake; and then came Oprah. If I was guilty of anything, it was being dazzled by Oprah: She was a beacon of light to me. But in my mind, I thought I handled the situation rather well, on a personal level, with no publicists involved. It seemed clear and sensible to me: I would do the *Today* show first, and then Oprah would show the wider story later.

But *politics got involved*. I believe the situation became a runaway train with supreme overreaction and a lot of emotion involved. If we had to do it all over again, both sides might act differently. Suffice to say, I was wounded and devastated, and felt the decision was unfair, particularly when Tom Touchet, then executive producer, told me I was "unanimously voted off the show." Unanimously voted off? Suddenly, I felt like a *Dancing with the Stars* castoff who couldn't master the mambo.

The pain and anger were overwhelming. The weeks that followed, as the press ate up the story, were very dark. The sensational headlines hurt: Seeing my name and the word "fired" in the same sentence stung. Enter steroid rage: All the psychological damage was inflamed by the massive quantities of antirejection steroids that I was ingesting every day.

I started going ballistic and having meltdowns in my house: I would scream until my throat was hoarse. I was vocal to begin with. Add steroids to that? Not pretty.

Old childhood issues began to resurface. In the Jewish religion, a boy becomes a man at age thirteen. The bar mitzvah is the traditional religious ceremony when a boy is called to the Torah to read and pray with a rabbi. A more modern twist is the afterparty; these are the male version of a sweet sixteen bacchanal, with themes like *Star Wars*, Disco Fever, or—my own theme—An Adventure in Shanghai. The custom is no gifts: Checks only. Generally, the money is intended to give the boy a start in life, but most boys I knew bought cars with their bar mitzvah money, or six thousand CDs, or invested heavily in Puma and video games. But in my case, my parents took the money to pay for practical matters, like my education and the kosher egg rolls at the party. I had always resented it, ever since I was thirteen, and in the weeks after I was fired, in my steroid rage, I decided to let my parents know.

Hysterical, I would scream at them: "Where is my bar mitzvah money? You stole it! I'm going to have you audited!"

While we were at it I decided to argue with them about other petty childhood issues, uncovering a decades-long resentment that I never knew I had. Why did I have to share a room with my sister until I was eight years old? Why was the house we grew up in so small? When I was screaming, beet red and furious, this all seemed completely rational.

My mother would just stand there and take my acid barrage. And then she would tiptoe off to her bedroom to cry. The nurse we had hired for the first few weeks to supervise my care, who was a godsend, and who really felt for my mother. She would come in after we fought and calm my mother down. "This is normal, it's not him speaking," the nurse would tell her. "It's the steroids."

"But it still really hurts," my mother would weep.

When I started screaming, I would watch my parents recoil as if my words had literally slapped their faces. But they just looked at me with great sympathy and kindness—and the more kindness they showed me, the more enraged I became. I *wanted* to spar. When you're on a steroid high, you want confrontation; but my parents were smart and intuitive, and they took it very stoically.

My heart breaks for my parents because they never knew who was going to show up at the table for dinner in those days. Was I going to be the steroid monster and snap and hiss at everything? Was I going to be depressed, or would they get Mr. Sunshine? It was *Guess Which Personality Is Coming to Dinne*r?

"You are making us feel like you don't want us here, but we're just here to help you!" my mother would tell me, as I seethed at her and my dad across the table. And when I came down from my drug trip I would realize what I'd done, and feel like the worst son in the world.

CHAPTER 8

Kidney Is the New Black

Dear friends, I'd like to introduce you to Annabelle.
Annabelle is the love child of
Miss Abby Finer and Mr. Steven Cojocaru.
This little bundle of love was born on January 14, 2005,
weighing approximately 5 ounces and
approximately 12 centimeters long.
Her color was a healthy deep pink, and she was in robust
health.

One of the serious, realistic risks for any kidney transplant patient is that their organ might not work. For the first six months to a year, a newly transplanted kidney is very vulnerable to rejection; it's the most delicate time, a period where you are on pins and needles, and the further out you are from surgery the better your chances are of keeping it long term. After a year, the percentage rate of people whose transplanted kidneys work for the rest of their lives is very high, but there's never any guarantee. The doctors had drilled this into me, but I decided I had a solution: I was going to name the kidney. How could anything possibly go wrong to a kidney named Annabelle, a name that sounded like the plucky heroine of a children's book?

Sometimes, I felt like Annabelle had a life of her own. I would read her passages from *Pat the Bunny* and talk to her: "You're going to grow up to be a fine, strong kidney, my little Belle! I promise I will never drink tap water, only the finest purified water from the artesian wells in the Yaqara Range of the Nakauvadra Mountains!" I quit the alcohol and cigarettes like the doctors told me to. I would rub her, a lot. Occasionally, I would direct my friends to greet Annabelle, just to keep her happy: "Here's my beautiful kidney. Say hello to my little apricot!"

So far, Annabelle seemed to be pleased with the attention. By the middle of February, a month after my surgery, I was well on the path to recovery. My twice-weekly visits to the doctor had grown easier and easier, and the results were uniformly positive: The kidney was functioning perfectly. I counted myself lucky. Everything was clicking, even though I was still extremely weak.

My doctor had insisted that I take at least two months off of work to recover, but by week five I was dying to go back. It was the middle of the awards season, and it was killing me that I would watch the red carpet parade from my couch. The People's Choice Awards, the SAG awards, the Grammy's—I missed them all. It was physically painful to not be a guest at the party, like having my arm hacked off.

On the morning after my transplant, in Cedars-Sinai, I had pronounced my recovery plans to Shari: "My goal is to work at the Oscars," I told her. But by mid-February, that still seemed like an unlikely proposition. I could barely walk up the stairs of my house, let alone sashay down the red carpet.

One morning, Linda Bell Blue, the executive producer of *Entertainment Tonight* and *The Insider*, called me to check in and see how I was doing. "You take as much time as you need to recover, but know that you are sorely missed," she said. She paused and added, "The Oscars is your thing. Do you think you could come back for it?"

I was on the phone with my doctor before we'd barely even hung up. "I want to be at the Oscars," I told him. "Even if I need an oxygen tent, a wheelchair, and a portable heart monitor on the carpet!"

"It's not going to happen," he told me. "You're still too susceptible to germs. You shouldn't leave your house."

I was devastated. The Oscars are the center of my universe. When I'm on the Oscars red carpet, I feel like the beaming bride: I have butterflies in my stomach. It's when I flash my megawatt, full-monty, patented Cojo smile, I mean, *all* my molars come out and my mouth is stretched to my ears. If you aren't giddy and excited as you face this night—the night of dreams, globally—and if you just phone it in, just going through the motions, then something is wrong. The Oscars are my yearly ritual, when I check in, ask myself: *Am I still excited? Not jaded? Can I still get goose bumps like a wide-eyed kid?* It's my bellwether, my compass. And this was the first time I would miss it in twelve years.

I called Linda back and told her the bad news. Her response was totally unexpected, and really quite magical. "OK, then, let's bring the red carpet to you," she said. "We'll just have you do the Oscars from your house."

My biorhythms nearly rocketed through my roof. If she'd been in the room, I would have taken off my mask and smooched her and spooned my mother's famous chocolate-chip cake into her mouth.

On the morning of February 27, a stampede of producers from *Entertainment Tonight* descended upon my house to turn my living room into an Oscars red carpet. They arrived with generators and satellite trucks, klieg lights, lighting grids, three different cameras, plus cameramen, lighting directors, audio engineers, grips, gaffers, makeup artists, and hair stylists. It was a full scale production: My neighbors probably thought we were making a porno film.

I had promised my doctor a crew of three: there had to be fifty people in my house. By Dr. Jordan's orders, the entire crew wore surgical masks. My dad became the unpaid production assistant: He was like a little kid, in his glory, bringing people water and coffee, peppering everyone with questions about what was going on. My mother was director of catering, producing mountains of home-made apple-cinnamon muffins from the kitchen.

For my grand return to the carpet, I was dressed to the nines in a vintage tux jacket with hand-painted silver slashes of glitter. I looked like a glamazon rock star—as long as you didn't look at the tuxedo pants, which had been picked up specially from the Big and Tall Store to accommodate my steroid-bloated stomach.

As the stars began to arrive, my producers patched me in to the Kodak Theater. I had a huge screen in my living room and on it, live, was the red carpet, just a mile south of me on Hollywood Boulevard. As soon as I saw the red carpet come up on the screen, there was no more pain: It just disappeared. The stars paraded by: Leo was soaking up the attention for *The Aviator*; Cate Blanchett glided past in lemon Valentino; and even though he was nominated for best actor for *Finding Neverland*, Johnny Depp forgot to wash his hair. The first time I saw Gwyneth Paltrow do a fashion twirl, an electrical current ran through me, all the way to my golden roots.

From my living room, I reported on the very best and worst dressed Oscars stars. I was patched in to Halle Berry. "Cojo! I hope you are doing well. I'm thinking about you," she said, with great emotion. I teared up. It was a moment with a capital M.

And then: Oprah, herself, came to the camera: Instead of Mo-hammed coming to the mountain, Mt. Everest had come to me. "You're in my prayer circle," she told me. I was floored. I could have floated all the way to the Kodak Theater.

It was the high of highs; glorious; it fed me. After everything I'd been through, the darkness of the steroids and getting fired, I was blinded by so much light. Despite the fact that I had had a transplant, that I was on pills to stay alive, that my life had been ruptured and put on spin cycle, here I was in my own home, with an earpiece in my head, and ten blocks away Oprah was wishing me me well! It was a turning point for me: I knew I was going to be OK no matter what. No matter what happened, if I was strapped down, if I was bedbound and missing every one of my organs, as long as my mouth worked I knew I would have a voice out there talking about train wrecks on the red carpet and who shouldn't be wearing a see-through lace slip dress by Dolce & Gabbana. My tongue had not been silenced. Even though stars with bruised egos had wanted to pull it out, step on it, run it over with their SUVs, the barbed tongue was alive and well.

For weeks, I'd barely been upright; but that day I stood before the cameras for eight hours, weak and aching, but so giddy with adrenaline that I barely noticed. What Linda had given me was monumental. She had brought me back into the world, motivated me to get better, to push myself. She was helping me grow beyond my disease. Sometimes it *is* mind over matter: You're in so much pain, but you push through it. Linda made me push myself, work, feel like part of the world again. She gave me a bigger gift than she'll ever know.

The other event that got me out of bed that March was my audience with Oprah. I saw this as a chance to tell my story to millions and hopefully have some kind of real impact. I was really fired up about promoting live kidney donors: There was such a severe kidney shortage in the world, and I didn't think people knew that the average person had the power to save somebody's life. It had worked for *me* in a dire situation. I wanted to scream it from the rooftops, galvanize people around the nation to open up their hearts. What better pulpit to shout from than Oprah's couch?

I'd bumped into Oprah at events for years: In my eyes, she was always larger than life, and her presence on the red carpet was electrifying. I like that she uses her show to inspire and change people. Even in our brief exchanges, she inspired me, too. Not long after I publicly announced that I was ill, I found myself interviewing her at a conference that Maria Shriver had organized. After the interview, Oprah pulled me aside, wanting to express her concern about my disease. It was, unexpectedly, one of the most emotional experiences of my life. She just looked me in the eyes, held my hands, and said two words: "Use it."

I took that to mean that I should use my illness to help other people; but as I thought about it some more, I also wondered whether she intended something more personal. "Use it"—did that mean that I should use this disease to better myself and grow into a stronger person, to become a more evolved and satisfied human being? In other words, to use it as a positive rather than a negative? As my illness progressed over the following year, I would come back to her words again and again.

By the end of March, I had been given a clean bill of health by Dr. Jordan and granted permission to fly to Chicago. My parents had returned to Montreal in early March, so I flew them, my sister Alisa, and Shari to Chicago. Abby flew in from New York, along with her family.

Being out in the real world for the first time since my surgery was surreal. I'd been in quarantine for so long—I hadn't had a normal life since October of 2004—that I felt like a different person, almost drunk with the sense of rebirth. Although my initial instincts had been to hide my disease, to keep it close to the hip, I was learning that the more you release it the healthier it is. I hoped that people could be inspired by my story. More and more, I was starting to experience a sense of kinship not just with other kidney patients, but with all people suffering from a major illness. It was like a catastrophe club: When someone came up to me and said "I have leukemia" or "I have breast cancer," everything seemed to stop for a moment. I would look in their eyes and know what they were going through; and they, too, would know how I felt.

Despite all this excitement, however, I was feeling under the weather. By the time I disembarked from the plane in Chicago, I felt slightly fluish, and my bones were hurting. The gallon of vitamin C–fortified orange juice that I swallowed didn't help. My family's plans for a gala celebratory dinner were shot. Instead, it was chicken soup delivered up to my hotel room.

Somehow I found the strength to address my wardrobe. In the week before my appearance, I had tried on every piece of clothing on the racks of Rodeo Drive. I was convinced that my wardrobe would somehow reveal something about this new person, this new *one-kidney wonder*. (For anyone who is counting, I originally had two "native" kidneys of my own which were covered with cysts. When my new transplant kidney was put in, the doctors didn't actually remove the native kidneys. Instead, I had three kidneys: two with the wires disconnected, so to speak, and one new, functioning kidney.) Up until that point, I had been working the raffish, rakish rock star look: To me, a suit was skin-tight jeans, rocker boots, and Jagger-esque scarves. Those binding two-button uniforms with the standard-issue tie and lace-up shoe were repulsive to me: It screamed Establishment. But for an occasion as momentous as going on Oprah, though, I decided I would wear a suit.

After attempting ten thousand shirt and tie and pocket square combinations, I had narrowed my options down to a handful. I took Polaroids of them all, brought the outfits to Chicago with me, and the night before my appearance Shari and I had a fashion show. I tried on each option over and over and over, until my friend cried for mercy. We finally settled on a pinstriped Gucci suit and Prada Chelsea boots, worn with a lavender gingham shirt and gold-lavender swirled tie. I wanted to be fashion forward, very chic and sleek. I was going for bloated James Bond: If 007 had a transplant and had been pumped full of the steroids until he was puffed out to the size of Anguilla, he would have looked like me.

I woke up at the break of dawn to prepare. My flu had grown worse during the night, and I was very very nervous. I'm not usually scared to go on TV, but this seemed larger than life: With my parents, sister, and Abby there, I felt the need to take care of everyone. That kind of stress used to be second nature to me, but I had been so worn down by the previous months, that it suddenly felt like too much. I was glad Shari was there to keep me upright.

As is the normal Canadian-Romanian custom, my family managed to stuff a dozen people in the limousine that took us to the *Oprah* show along with a deli counter set up with steamed cabbage, cabbage on ice, cabbage a la mode, grilled cabbage and California roll cabbage. We were all in our Sunday best, as if we were going to cotillion. Because we are Jewish, Barbra Streisand has, by default, always been our spiritual leader; but that day, she was forever replaced by Oprah.

Backstage at *Oprah* is beautiful. I've been through many backstages in my life and most look like they are leftover from vaudeville days. *Oprah's* backstage was modern, busy, and comfortable. Since I had already done my own hair and makeup, Oprah's staff put themselves to work on my mother and Shari instead, in case the camera panned over to them. My sister, who is the love child of Estée Lauder and Max Factor, a girl who used crayons as eyeshadow back in kindergarden, was already made up with enough sparkle, glitter, and eyeshadow for a reunion of Destiny's Child. I'm sure she got up at 1:00 a.m. because her hair was pressed, starched, her makeup immaculate, her nails impeccable, her outfit perfect.

My troop went into the audience, I got a final powder, and I was sent into a green room to wait by myself. While I waited, Oprah aired the pre-taped material her crew had shot of me, the morning of my surgery. A production assistant told me how I would be cued and where I would walk, and then, in those final moments backstage I was overcome with emotion. *I survived this!* I thought. *I'm alive! Seven months ago I was at the precipice of darkness, and here I am.* I felt triumphant. My heart was pounding as I walked out on stage. I heard the audience clapping and cheering, felt Oprah hugging me, and I knew that people were pulling for me.

Abby came onstage with me and received the heroes' welcome, as she should. I felt she deserved a twenty-one gun salute. Nothing is a big enough thank you for the person who has done the ultimate sacrifice and loved you so wholeheartedly that they would give you one of their organs.

As I sat onstage with Oprah, I told her how I was feeling. "I see myself as a better person in so many ways," I told her. "I found out I am incredibly positive: I'm Pippi Longstocking. Abby gave me life, she saved my life, bottom line. I've been bathed in love. I see nothing but good. Friends and family have come together to get me through this, and it's made me a better person. I call this a gift."

It was powerful and beautiful, and all too soon, it was all over. And then my family arrived to meet us backstage. Wild-eyed and pumped-up, my family came to worship at the shrine of Oprah. My mother cornered her and began talking to her about the color of a dress she wore to the Emmy's ten years earlier; my sister was yapping in her ear about Oprah's gorgeous eyeshadow; my father was snapping photographs; and I was cringing. But Oprah was so kind and warm and gracious, aware of what this meant to my parents. Indeed, in my parents' house, over the mantel, in the place of honor, now sits the gold-framed photograph of them with Oprah; my graduation portrait has been relegated to the bathroom next to the porcelain tissue box holder.

We were supposed to go out that night to celebrate, but I was still feeling under the weather, so instead, we had a pajama party, with onion rings and spaghetti and meatballs and cake delivered up to my room. We stayed up until two in the morning rehashing the day's events. That day felt like a resolution, for all of us. I've always been a dreamer who believes in happy endings, just like you see in the movies. It's a sickness I suffer from, a belief in fairy tales with a beginning, middle, and end. This, for me, was *my* happy ending, with a pretty bow on top. I saw the last seven months as my own personal Bette Davis saga: the strife, then the illness, the soap opera of getting fired, the humiliation and the headlines, and then my miraculous return, he's alive and kicking, going on *Oprah*, cut to credits, the end, upbeat music and ride off to Sunset Boulevard. I truly believed that was it, without a doubt.

CHAPTER 9

Requiem for Annabelle

I had returned home to Los Angeles expecting not just to have a good life: I expected a *fabulous* life. I was going to pick up right where I left off seven months earlier, put my life back on like a perfectly cut French suit. Everything would happen according to my master plan, no restrictions, no change of habits. It was suffer the transplant, go on *Oprah*, and you're cured—almost like Oprah was a shaman who had given me the final healing I needed.

The whole production line was beginning again. Shoes were being polished, outfits were put together, vats of peroxide were being readied, and my dance card was starting to fill. There were premieres to attend. I penciled in *Sahara*, which was premiering on April 4, 2005. I was hoping that Penelope would make her grand entrance on a camel, and that just by shaking Matthew's hand my man-boob pecs would harden. I had front-row tickets to see U2 at the Staples Center in early April, and I'd been obsessing over the concert for months. *Bono was going to spit on me!* In my house, it was U2 twenty-four hours a day.

But the cold that I'd come down with in Chicago wasn't going away; in fact, it was getting worse. The doctor had told me that since I was such a recent transplantee, still very vulnerable, that I should call him even if I got the beginnings of a bunion. But I blew it off: *It's just a cold*, I rationalized. *I'll be fine.*

But by the morning of the U2 concert, I was so weak that I couldn't get out of bed; I alternated between extreme chills and soaring fevers. My entire body was taken over by severe aches, from head to toe. I was struck ill all of a sudden, as if my lights had been punched out. I had blackouts, flashes, and strange dreams of dancing kidneys, stethoscopes that came alive like snakes, and orderlies with axes. It was time to send up a smoke signal to Dr. Jordan.

"You have to come in immediately for a blood test," he insisted.

I gave the U2 tickets away to a friend who had to physically tear them out of my viselike grip. And then I drove myself to Cedars-Sinai, hoping that I'd get an antibiotic and a nothing-to-worry-about diagnosis from Dr. Jordan.

Dr. Jordan took my blood and sent me home, promising to call later with the results. I came back just in time to get into my jammies, pop a sleeping pill, and catch the last twenty minutes of *The View*. I was going to sleep away my worries for the rest of the afternoon. I was in REM 72, on a whitewater river rafting trip in the Congo with my "buds" Aaron Eckhart and Tom Brady, when the phone rang. It was Jenny from Dr. Jordan's office. "I'm sorry, but your kidney numbers are really elevated," she said. "Dr. Jordan needs you to have a kidney biopsy. Why don't you take an hour to get your stuff together, and then I'm going to need to check you in to the hospital. You'll be doing a biopsy first thing tomorrow."

No, no, no. I was supposed to get the kidney transplant and then live happily ever after. I had already fought so much in such a short time that I hadn't even had a chance to catch my breath and process what had happened—and now, I had to deal with even more? It didn't seem right. But this was the part of the conversation with Dr. Jordan that I had tuned out, the fine print that explained about the complications and the risks and the horror stories about kidneys not lasting.

There is no easy way to really confirm if your body is rejecting a transplanted kidney: the doctors can't just draw blood or have you pee in a cup. The only way to tell what's going on is to biopsy the kidney and look at a piece of it under a microscope. This is how a biopsy works. You get The Call that your blood tests have come back and your kidney's creatinine number is high. (Your creatinine number is a measurement of the function of your kidney and how well it is filtering out the toxins in your body.) This might just be the result of the toxic drugs that you're taking, but there's a chance that you might be rejecting. It's every kidney patient's nightmare, the Big R. So pack your bags: You're going to be spending a night in the hospital and getting a biopsy.

You check in to the third floor of Cedars-Sinai and are assigned a day bed, one of a dozen tiny little cubicles in a big room. There you are, back in the hospital again, and you are feeling traumatized. This is not a little thing: It's a *thing*. As you undress, your heart is sinking, you're asking yourself, *Am I going to come out of the hospital alive? Will I go home without a kidney?*

You aren't allowed to eat. If your biopsy is scheduled for the afternoon and runs late, you might not have had a bite since dinner the previous evening. You lie there, in a hospital gown, waiting, hungry. Eventually, your bed is wheeled in to a small operating room. It's serious enough that there's a whole team there: two kidney doctors, a handful of nurses, the ultrasound technician, the pathologist. They give you a Valium to relax you and then the ultrasound technician looks around for a spot on your stomach. And then—*Whap!* They stab you with a gigantic needle, like a staple gun, pierce your stomach and pull a piece of your kidney out. The pathologist examines the sample; and then, frequently, they'll say "I don't have enough." Which means they are going to go back and do the whole thing again.

Even if the biopsy is successful, you can't just say *ta-ta*. You have to stay motionless for fear of bleeding, and you'll have to stay over-night in the hospital. If the doctors think that your body might be rejecting the kidney you'll be injected with a massive dose of ste-roids. Steroids cause you to retain water, so you can imagine what happens: You bloat up until your face is so swollen and distorted that you look like a Bundt cake.

I had four biopsies in the months after my kidney transplant. What the doctors finally discovered was that I had contracted the polyomavirus in my kidney. Annabelle had been infected with a very common bug, one of a multitude of bacterium that humans host in their bodies that, with a *healthy* immune system, are usually killed off every day. In a normal body the polyomavirus would be insig-nificant and undetectable. But once it got into my body, with my compromised immune system, it flared up and came to life, like a dormant animal waking up.

I don't know why I was so cavalier when my doctors told me what was wrong in mid-April. "What do I need to take to get rid of it?" I asked. I felt medically cocky: I'd survived a transplant! Surely I could knock out a little virus.

"No," Dr. Jordan said. "It's a little more complicated than that."

By the end of April, one of the doctors that was monitoring my kidney—Dr. Moss—was predicting that the polyomavirus was going to kill Annabelle. "This is very serious, this virus," he told me. "It's very likely you will lose your kidney. You need to prepare yourself for that."

But I refused to believe it. In a very polite way, I told him to fuck off and die. I wasn't losing my kidney! The thought of losing this precious kidney was too painful, too devastating to even consider. How could I go through all that again?

The fighter inside me came alive: Sure, I was devastated and hurt and scared by what he'd told me, but something bigger inside me said, *No way, no way, this is not going to happen, he is being alarmist.*

And even if Dr. Moss was pessimistic, Dr. Jordan was still encouraging. "You are going to survive this!" he told me. "It's tough, it's going to be a fight, but we are not giving up. We are going to do everything we can to save this kidney."

In May, Dr. Jordan put me on an extreme course of IVIG—the equivalent of flooding your body with a very powerful cocktail of proteins that fight immune disorders—to kill off the polyomavirus. Every few weeks for eight hours at a time, I would have to lie in the hospital bed with a needle in my arm, as IV fluids dripped slowly into my bloodstream. I would will myself to get better, praying until I was cross-eyed from the effort. But my creatinine numbers still kept creeping higher, until I was practically living in Cedars-Sinai again.

Throughout this ordeal, from the moment I got diagnosed, through all the bumps in the road—the trials and tribulations, the perils of Pauline—humor and imagination were my firing squad. They were my salvation. When you are in a hospital, steeped in tragedy and surrounded by the stench of disease, there's nothing more potent than escaping with your daydreams. Imagination was my satellite TV: It could take me away better than any DVD. When I was in my daydreams, I wasn't sick. It was a reprieve.

. . . *"Who's the first in the congo line?!" I blast through the halls of Cedars-Sinai: "Get up everybody! Grab your piña coladas: Cojo says it's time to stop being sick! We're having a luau!!"*

I'm dancing my way across the sixth floor in a sarong, singing "Tiny Bubbles" as I strum on my ukulele. Behind me, all the nurses are hula dancing and wearing leis made of Dixie cups. The chief of surgery has ripped off his lab coat and is blowing bubbles, which bounce off the dialysis machines and fill the air. Chocolate syrup is pouring through all the IVs, and jelly beans are flooding out of the air vents.

The patients have come to the doorways of their rooms, dragging their heart monitors behind them. They spill out into the hallway, beaming, and begin to dance. Mrs. Leibowitz, a sixty-five-year-old liver transplantee, flips her bedpan upside down and turns it into a bongo. A trio of congenital heart failure patients are performing a chorus line of high kicks.

Behind the nurses station, Sol, an octogenarian kidney recipient, and his hunched-over friend Manny, a lung cancer patient, are rolling gigantic medical marijuana spliffs. "Duuude, this is the good stuff," Manny says. "Ja, man. Crank up the Bob Marley!" Sol replies.

The doctors come flooding into the halls, shouting, "You've all been cured! None of you are sick anymore! Go home!" Confetti rains down from the ceiling as the cheering patients form a parade and skip straight out the door. . .

. . . In my fantasies, I was the pied piper of joy and merriment. I could turn Cedars-Sinai into a Carnival Cruise. But in real life, I wasn't in the driver's seat. I was at the mercy of a never-ending stream of doctors, nurses, orderlies, technicians, and professional blood-taking vampires. And the news kept getting worse.

By June it was clear that the IVIG drips weren't working. I was living and dying by my creatinine numbers. I called them the Nielsen ratings: My friends from *Entertainment Tonight* would call every day and ask, "How are the numbers?" In most people, the creatinine numbers are less than 1.5. Mine were 5s and 6s, and every day the doctors were coming in with the bad news that the number was going up and up. Annabelle was dying.

Once again, I cut myself off from all my friends and family and kept the news about my impending kidney failure to myself. All the hard work I'd done—stay the course, be positive, fight the fight—went out the window. Weighing most heavily on me was the thought of Abby. I felt so sorry for her, as if I had let her down. Her sacrifice had been so tremendous, and, tragically, it had all been for naught. Our kidney was failing, but I felt like it was me who was failing her. I couldn't tell her. I didn't have the heart or the guts to pick up the phone and tell her that I was losing her precious kidney. Instead, I asked my mother to call her for me. It would take months for me to finally look Abby in the eyes again.

Maybe I could have done more? Maybe I shouldn't have flown to Oprah so soon after my transplant? When I started feeling ill, maybe I shouldn't have waited a day or two to call the doctor? I internalized it and made it my fault.

There is a kind of sadness where there are no words. I spent a lot of time alone in the dark. I didn't want the lights on. I drifted in and out of consciousness, thinking about Abby. I felt flattened.

In near-kidney failure, I had to move in to Cedars-Sinai for full-time care. When my kidney numbers careened to a near-lethal 8, my team of doctors came to see me. I knew the minute they opened the door and piled into the room: Their pallor and somber posture said it all. The kidney was coming out, and I was going to have to go on dialysis.

"We're going to take this one day at a time," Dr. Jordan told me. He went into positivity overdrive: "We're going to take out this kidney. We're going to put you on dialysis and get you better. As soon as the polyomavirus is cleaned out of your system, in the next few months, we can start to look for a new transplant."

I didn't hear him, because I was too busy shrieking and hyperventilating. I felt like I'd been struck by the Gods: Not only was I losing a loved one's gift, but I was going to have to be kept alive by a machine. I was hyperventilating as the doctors explained to me what dialysis would mean: Four hours of blood filtering, three times a week, to clear out all the toxins that would build up in my blood when I had no kidneys anymore. I'd already heard stories about dialysis, about how after a session you feel drained of all life. No wonder I feared it to the marrow: I couldn't even say the word. It was only to be referred to as the Big D, just like the hospital was only to be called The Hotel.

The quiet rage rose up in me. "I can't take this right now," I said, with a hiss. "I'm done with all this kidney stuff. I'm done. Can all of you just leave me alone for a while? Please, just get out of here."

As soon as they left, when the coast was clear and their clicking heels had faded off into the distance, I threw a party. I was the only guest: It was an all-night pity party. I repeated Dr. Jordan's words over and over in my brain. If I didn't have the kidney removed, if I didn't go on dialysis, I would die. It was black and white. I couldn't do that to my parents. The sensible adult inside me gave me a lecture: *You can be petulant or stubborn*, it said, *but this hold-your-breath-till-your-face-turns-blue thing just isn't working. You're not ready to die by any stretch of the imagination. You have to stay alive. That's it. That's all.*

I picked up the phone and called Shari. It was 2:00 a.m. The minute I heard her voice, everything broke and I started gutturally sobbing. "It's just been a terrible day," I cried. "I am so scared and so alone."

The next morning, I called my parents and told them that it was Tragedy, the Sequel. They had to fly down to Los Angeles so they could be with me and mourn the passing of the hope that we had nourished with all our hearts. The kidney was coming out. I was going on dialysis.

CHAPTER 10

Diva Does Dialysis

This is what my day planner says for the last week of June 2005. Tuesday, June 21—Pick up Vicodin; Call Regina to set up dialysis. Call Dr. Jordan. Wednesday, June 22—Order antiobiotics. Call agent. Jimmy Choo party at the Cartier boutique. Thursday, June 23—Party at Teddys at the Roosevelt Hotel. Friday, June 24: Pick up Vicodin.

On Monday, June 27, there is only a blank page. That day, I had my new kidney taken out.

I had to go back to the hospital, on dialysis the morning after my doctors delivered the bad news—a few days before my nephrectomy (the medical term for the removal of a kidney). I was completely by myself. I could have reached out to numerous people, but there was no way anyone was going to see me at one of the ugliest moments of my life. I could never face the humiliation of friends seeing me this downed, this felled. The only people I wanted around me were my parents, but they were still on an airplane en route to me.

I stayed up all night before my first dialysis session, growing more and more furious that this was happening to me as the hour approached. I felt like I was waiting for my own execution. The machine was rolled into my room at Cedars-Sinai at the break of dawn:

it was so enormous that it could barely fit through the door. It was creaky and ancient, with flaking metal and old knobs, and it looked like the first dialysis machine ever invented. I practically thought the nurse was going to jump on a bicycle to generate it's power.

The nurse went through a long series of preparations, taking out tools and needles and tubes, while I stared daggers at her. "They've made a mistake," I spit at her. "Stop. Get the *hell* out of here." I've never hated anyone as much in my life.

She smiled through her teeth; mine wasn't the first bedside horror movie she'd watched before. She was Miss Tough Love 2005. "Well," she said. "If I don't do it now, I'll have to come back later. Your choice."

This enraged me even more. I was semi-psychotic, wild-eyed, and fuming. In my head, I was battling the desire to be violent, throw fits and tantrums like a child; but reluctantly the adult voice said *Get over yourself. Just do it, and grit your teeth.*

I looked at her, feeling utterly defeated. "All right," I said.

Hemodialysis works by withdrawing the blood very slowly out of your body through a catheter in your neck that works like a direct plug into your veins. The blood flows into the dialysis machine, where a special filter filled with a spongelike fluid takes out all the wastes and extra liquids from the blood and then returns it slowly to your body through another tube. The machine monitors your blood pressure and maintains healthy levels of chemicals like potassium and sodium. It is, basically, a giant electronic kidney.

For the next four hours, as I did my first dialysis treatment, bile oozed from my pores. My loathing for the nurse and for the world at large didn't let up for one second. You would think with my blood being cleansed I would have felt like life was being put back into me; but it was quite the contrary. It was more like the life was being sucked out of me. I lay there fading in and out of consciousness; but every time I opened up my eyes and saw the nurse with that machine, my jaw would clench and I would come alive again: *Her!* She was the focal point for my venom. As each hour passed in the abyss, my body may have been physically weakening, but my mind, fueled by hatred, was sharp as a tack. Nothing could stop me from plotting her slow, hideous demise: I imagined snakes slithering out of the machine, biting her with their fangs, their poison sucking away at her central nervous system.

My parents arrived breathless from the airport two days later, clutching the Samsonite luggage that they'd gotten for a sexy weekend tryst in Niagara Falls in the early 1970s. When they walked in the room to find me hooked up to the dialysis machine, their faces froze. I watched as they tried to gain their composure, but it was too much. My mother caressed my forehead with her hand, and my father kept asking, "How are you doing?" but their eyes couldn't help darting back to the machine.

We sat there, all afternoon, going through the motions. My mother couldn't bake a chocolate-chip cake to fix this one. Finally, we began to talk about the reality that my kidney was going to be removed in two days. It was over. And we began to go through the mourning process—we were sitting shiva for Annabelle.

After a day of this, my mother snapped out of it: it was enough bleakness, enough bathing in the dark. She made a special announcement: "No more grieving." She had watched me fading away and something in her finally decided, "I can't let him go into this with all of us in such bad shape."

My mother launched her full-scale Operation Sunshine mission.

She summoned my friend Linda: "Bring Stinky over immediately." I hadn't seen my dog in two months—while I went in and out of the hospital, he had been living with Linda and Steve, their daughter Sophie, and their two poodles, Lucky and Chelsea. Living without him was like having a hole in my heart: I was pining for him. That afternoon, I went down to the hospital's outdoor plaza, in my bathrobe and slippers and PJs, with hair that hadn't seen a comb in a week. I sat on a bench in the garden, next to the lung cancer patients who were smoking (the hospital had generously provided ashtrays for them: I'm surprised they didn't have a crack-smoking section), and waited for my dog to arrive.

I don't know what fences Linda jumped, but she somehow smuggled Stinky into that plaza. It was like a slow-motion scene out of *Love Story:* I could have sworn I heard violins. Stinky saw me, leaped into my arms, and then my Maltese started howling like I'd never heard him howl before. My heart exploded: It was a major reunion.

That night, my mother decided that we were going to have a celebration in my room. We were all starving: I wasn't keeping food down, my parents hadn't eaten in weeks from anxiety. But mostly, we were hungry to be repaired, hungry for a respite from our suffering.

So we had an in-room pizza party. This was a big no-no. On hemodialysis, I was on a very strict diet. I couldn't eat tomatoes, avocados, or bananas, for fear of getting too much potassium in my blood; and milk and cheese were restricted for fear of a phosphorus overdose. I was being fed egg white omelettes—exactly three egg whites. Even my water was measured out, drop by drop.

But I felt like the misery I was enduring had given me a Get Out of Jail Free card: I just didn't care anymore. I had received my baby, sweet, keeping-me-alive kidney in January and here I was in June, and it was gone, poof. All that time, I'd been the model patient: I'm not one for rules, but I'd done everything to the letter. Not anymore. That night, it was everything be damned. If I was going to go down I was going to go down in a blaze of carbs and dairy and sugar and nicotine.

In my bathrobe, I crawled my way to the elevator, and snuck down to the hospital plaza to smoke one last illicit cigarette. Wheezing and short of breath, I inhaled an entire pack. Then I went back upstairs, guzzled a liter of diet soda, devoured a pizza on my own, had two heaping pieces of chocolate cake.

I felt sick afterward: My stomach had expanded, and I was bloated and depressed. Instead of a celebration, that meal suddenly felt like the Last Supper.

I woke up after the nephrectomy with a flood of thoughts racing through my head: Once again, it was the pain, the depression, the sense of defeat. But one thought kept floating to the surface until I became fixated on it: What had happened to Annabelle? What had the surgeons done with the kidney when they took it out? With all that we went through, had she just been tossed away in a trash bag? Was she in a Dumpster? Was she in the Cedars-Sinai incinerator at this very moment?

I called Dr. Jordan in, barely coherent. I realized I was crying. "Dr Jordan," I said. "What happened to Annabelle?"

He looked at me, confused. "Who?"

"Annabelle! My kidney! What did you do with my kidney when you took her out?"

He smiled, very gently. "The kidney has gone to pathology, where it will be studied. We'll be using it to learn about the nature of this virus for future transplantees."

I was strangely comforted by this fact, and in the days to come, when I felt like I had hit bottom, I would sometimes think about that. The kidney had gone to a good place: It wasn't for naught. I could see the bigger picture. In my mind, Annabelle deserved a Nobel Peace Prize for scientific medical research; I was already planning the oufit for the ceremony in Stockholm. Margiela, I thought.

Another fashion miracle: I'd made it to the Hospital Ward A-list at last. Getting a kidney taken out had landed me on the Club Floor. Lindsay, schmindsay; Britney—whatever: Some divine intervention had decided I was getting to hop past the star-u-tants and net the ultimate in superstardom. I had landed in the Audrey Hepburn Memorial Suite. It seemed darkly poetic that fashion-obsessed me was in the same room where this style icon, a woman I had always worshipped, had spent her final days battling cancer.

I went home with my parents at the end of June without a single functioning kidney to my name, and with the address of an outpatient dialysis center in Beverly Hills in my day planner. This dialysis center would be my new second home, a place I would be visiting three times a week, four hours a visit, until I finally found a new kidney to replace the one that I'd just lost. If that never happened, I'd be coming to this center for the rest of my life.

At least it would be in a good neighborhood. It was right in the middle of Robertson Boulevard, Los Angeles' shopping nirvana, kitty-corner from Kitson, where Paris Hilton and her friends blow their trust funds; and the organic juice bar where you can stop in for a $12 mango-wheatgerm smoothie with a boost of ginkgo biloba. I thought that the dialysis center would be like an annex of the Ivy: I'd get a $30 chopped salad along with some clean new blood.

I walked into the dialysis center with a virgin eye, expecting—because of its location—muted lighting, chandeliers, zebra rugs, and gorgeous wallpaper, maybe some Lalique crystal figurines of kidneys. What I saw was worse than anything I could have dreamed of—and when I dream dark things, it's *Night of the Living Dead* meets *Apocalypse Now*. If I'd thought dialysis was bad at the hospital, that was the La Prairie Spa at the Beverly Hills Hotel—the one downstairs with the beautiful peach damask wallpaper—compared to this.

This place felt like a triage center in a war zone. It was one enormous room, with dozens of sick people sitting in old torn La-Z-Boy chairs, attached to machines. The place reeked of illness and medicine and blood. The dialysis machines made cold, computerized noises—beeping and clicking and rattling and buzzing. And everywhere I turned, patients—many elderly and very fragile—were moaning. An ambulance was ominously parked at the front entrance, with paramedics at the ready, waiting for someone to collapse. Adding to the grisly scene were the nurses, who wore paper hazmat suits with plastic shields. Standing in the doorway, it felt to me like the world had come to an end, and I was in a biological warfare recovery center.

I was seeing all this through the eyes of someone who had been sheltered. Up until that point I had been alone in my hospital room with no one to measure myself against. Suddenly, I was surrounded by other kidney patients, and it was horrifying. I've learned since that people who are on dialysis long-term grow comfortable with the process: It's a fact of life for them. They build a little community, they get to know the nurses, make friends over the years, and start kidney cliques. But I didn't see the other dialysis patients as comrades yet; I didn't want to even make eye contact with them, because I didn't want to be one of them. I was in so much denial, so angry, that I needed to divorce myself from all this. So I put my blinders on and refused to speak to anybody. If someone smiled at me, I looked the other way. If I opened a crack in the door, I was afraid I'd be sucked in.

"This is the most horrible place I have seen in my entire life, bar none," I told my mother, as we walked through the center to my assigned machine. I clung to her like I was a barnacle. "I can't do this."

This Romanian rock of Gibraltar held my hand while the nurse was hooking me up to the machine. My mother sat there for four hours, stroking my face, massaging my hands, as I slipped in and out of consciousness. I couldn't read because I was seeing double: trying to read *W* magazine felt like tackling *The Brothers Karamazov* in its original Russian. I was too tired to do anything but sleep and watch the blood flow hypnotically back and forth through the tubes until it put me in a trance. The smell of chemicals and blood was over-whelming, the worst kind of medicinal smell. I felt as if my body's circuits had been fried, and my electrical system was going nuts. My feet burned like they were on fire, I had indescribable aches, and my body seemed to separate completely from my mind.

As I lay there, feeling my worst, I suddenly thought of my last va-cation in Paris. Of course, I went shopping and bought every French designer label. I bought a beret. I almost bought a jockstrap with a French flag on it. When I walked down the cobblestone streets in my Lanvin boots the smell of piping hot croissants wafted through my remodeled nostrils. I practically bathed in café au lait. I lost myself for hours in vintage jewelry stores on the Left Bank; in the loveliest park in Paris, the Place des Vosges in the funky Marais; and in the inspiring sight of older French women on the streets, carrying them-selves so elegantly, the epitome of chic with their carefully coiffed hair and their artfully arrayed silk scarves.

I lay there and remembered sitting in the front row of Chanel Couture during Paris fashion week, remembered going to a wild party for a YSL fragrance called NU, where a human fishbowl was full of seminude models, remembered my pilgrimage to the memorial for Princess Diana and getting lost in the Luxembourg Gardens. The beauty and glamour of Paris, for a moment, took the pain away.

But as I sat plugged in to a dialysis machine, I suddenly feared that I'd never get back to Paris. I was going to be a prisoner for the rest of my life. I would be chained to this machine, living on pills, so sick that travel would be out of the picture. I turned to my mother: "Do you think I'll ever go to Paris again?" I asked.

"Of course, you are going to go to Paris," she told me. "You're going to get a new kidney, the doctor said your life is going to go back to normal. I promise you, you'll go back to France."

The last time she had been in Paris, she told me, was when she was emigrating to Canada with my father, in the early 1960s. They were poor, staying in a slum neighborhood, and they could barely afford a baguette. Talk about perspective. Here I was on Robertson Boulevard, where at that very minute Beverly Hills princesses were dropping a thousand dollars on rhinestone flipflops and leather halter tops while their mothers with swollen lips and barely-recovered brow lifts were drinking mint juleps at the Ivy, pissing away time. But in the dialysis center, only yards away, people were being kept alive on machines. That point was not lost on me then, and it's still not lost on me. To this day, when I drive by that corner my heart drops. I think about who is in there, that very second, trying to survive, watching the blood run out of their body, while Mrs. Synthetic Beak is getting wedge heels at Diavolina.

When Shari returned to Montreal after my first transplant, we had planned a summer vacation in Los Angeles together. All spring, it had been the thing that kept my spirits up. In my delusional mind, my little kidney Annabelle was going to be in perfect shape six months after my transplant: I was going to be healed and slim again, my hair would be highlighted and my life would be jolly. Everything would be fine, and Shari and I would have a magic week of spa visits and shopping.

I had no idea that would not be the case. When Shari arrived in early July, I was at my absolute weakest physically since this whole illness had begun. I hadn't yet discovered that I was being overmedicated by my psychiatrist; I was doing hemodialysis three times a week; I was still recovering from the nephrectomy; and as a result I was aching, suffering from unbearable nausea and dizziness. I was a shell of myself.

Shari took over babysitting duties. All that week, she washed and folded my unmentionables, sacrificed her Chanel nail polish scrubbing my bathtub, took Stinky for walks, and prepared me chef salads with her homemade Roquefort dressing (which truth be told, tasted like brake fluid). She drove me to my hemodialysis appointments and wasn't embarrassed to be seen with me even though the fashion maven had become a fashion disaster: It was July and hot, but I was still wearing January's hip-hop New York Street look, a black velour tracksuit. It was very *Sopranos* meets Missy Elliot: all that was missing was the big gold chains. With no ventilation, I was overheated in that outfit, but I was too sick and depressed to care. Shari would sit there with me and hold my hand as I did the dialysis. Together, we would joke about how we were going to start a nail polish line that replicated the color of the blood running through the tubes.

My one goal for that week was to take Shari to the Louis Vuitton store to buy a purse. The way an old grandma offers you hard candy, I offer my girlfriends handbags: I have a hard time saying "I love you," so my way of showing affection is Fendi. Purses are my Hallmark card, my currency. And in the middle of my delirium I had promised Shari a handbag as a thank-you for being there, for taking care of my parents, for getting on a plane every time there was a problem. Besides, Shari is a Pavlovian dog. If you wave a handbag in front of her you can get anything out of her. She would trek across the Serengeti for a tote.

Every morning, I woke up hoping that that would be the day that I felt well enough to make the pilgrimage to Vuitton. Every day, it took all the energy I could muster just to make it to dialysis. Finally, at four o'clock on Shari's last day in town, I roused myself from my fevered daze. "We're going to go," I announced. Sweating profusely, I took off the velour tracksuit and put on jeans, a white shirt, and a blazer. My feet were burning from the dialysis, I could barely move, but I'd promised her a bag and I was going to make it happen.

When we walked in the door of Louis Vuitton, minutes before it closed for the day, I was dragging my feet. My stomach was so distended that the buttons were popping off my shirt; I had somehow managed to squeeze myself into a size 38 waist jeans that were viciously boring into my tender abdomen. Shari was barely suppressing her inner wild hyena: She was panting and drooling all over the purse counter.

Suddenly, the smell of leather opened my nasal passages. My pounding headache vanished as I fondled a $1,770 Vuitton logo pet carrier. It was monograms, monograms, everywhere: I was hypnotized. Shari was trying to get my attention and show me bags, but it was too late: I was gone. In my monogrammed delirium, I abandoned Shari at the purse counter and raced through the store, my heart pounding, as I touched everything: scarves, shoes, billfolds, umbrellas, iPod holders. As I rubbed myself against the mannequins, it hit me that—other than the hospital gift shop—I hadn't been in a store in months.

That shopping trip, I realized, wasn't just for Shari—it was also for me. When you are sick, you become so grateful of anything that gives you a flash of your healthy life. I needed to be in a retail store again and hear the humming meditative sound of credit card machines. I'd longed to be around avarice again, with all those materialistas under one roof, clawing over hugely overpriced luxury products. I couldn't have been happier if I had had an audience with the Dalai Lama at the Louis Vuitton boutique in Tibet.

Dialysis still wasn't getting any easier; in fact, it was growing more unbearable every visit. I thought of spending the rest of my life in that place and wanted to throw myself under a bus on Sunset Boulevard.

I called Dr. Jordan and told him I couldn't do it anymore. "I can't cope with this," I told him. "I know what I'm capable of and not capable of. Are there any other options than going three times a week?"

Dr. Jordan considered my question. "Yes," he said. "Right now you are doing hemodialysis. But there's another option called peritoneal dialysis. You do that kind at home. You have to do it every day; but I think you would be a really good candidate for it." While hemodialysis filters your blood outside of your body in a machine, he explained, peritoneal dialysis filters your blood inside your body.

If I chose to do this, I would have a permanent tube inserted into my stomach, and every night, while I slept, a small machine called a cycler would pump my stomach full of a dextrose solution that would clean my blood and then drain all the waste fluid out. Over the course of a night, the machine would do two of these "exchanges," at four hours per exchange, and in the morning I would have two bags of body waste to empty.

Not every kidney patient is a candidate for peritoneal dialysis for a variety of reasons subject to their physical condition. It also isn't recommended for everyone, since you're doing it yourself at home and it requires extreme diligence and responsibility. There are a lot of risks and no margin for error. But I was willing to do anything to make my escape from the dialysis center.

"Sign me up," I told him.

"I have to warn you," Dr. Jordan continued. "Your stomach will be very distended. Everything gets pumped into your belly, and you will bloat like nothing you've ever seen. And if you aren't extremely careful about being sterile, you can get peritonitis, which is an extremely lethal infection. And because you won't be in a hospital you won't be near doctors who can help you immediately if there's a problem."

I didn't hesitate. "Yes, no question about it. Anything to save me from going back to that place," I said.

But my other doctor, Dr. Moss, was totally opposed to the idea of peritoneal dialysis. "You've been talking about your vanity this whole time," he told me when I called him to discuss it. "With peritoneal your stomach will retain liquid and you will bloat. There is no way around it. You will blow up."

"You've got to be kidding me," I said to him. "You're now my stylist? Come on. I've been living in purgatory, and now I have a chance to get out. I don't give a crap about my vanity now. I don't care if I'm the size of the Beverly Center. Right now, this is a godsend. I'll deal with the rest later." And then I "fired" him for being the Grinch Who Stole Kidney.

I was learning that doctors are not divine beings like my mother had always said. Doctors weren't *always* right. Instead, I had found a great empowerment in the midst of my disease: Sometimes *I* was right.

CHAPTER 11

One Day I'll See My Privates Again

When I started the Big D, my doctors warned me that I would retain water and should expect a little weight gain. Weight gain? What happened to me was more than packing on a few pounds: No one warned me that I'd get stuck in the doorway of Casa del Ratner. By the fall of 2005, I had ballooned to 220 pounds.

It took me a while to realize that I had gotten so enormous. There were little, very subtle hints: The fact that I had to move up five sizes in jeans. My new potbelly, which looked like I'd swallowed a watermelon. My thick swollen ankles. Even the shirts, which I now had to buy in a size 17.5, should have been a giveaway. But in my distorted brain I thought that if I could get my hair blown out and wear a dark baggy jacket to cover my distended stomach, I'd appear slim.

At the end of August I did my big comeback interview on *Entertainment Tonight*. I nearly flatlined when I saw myself on that screen: I was so bloated, so loaded down with double chins, that I didn't recognize myself. Whoever that person was on television, he was a junior rhino, and not even a raw silk Comme des Garçons blazer could hide that distorted body.

My vanity came flooding back with a vengeance.

People were very kind. "I saw the interview," people would say. They would hesitate, and look at me with pitying eyes. "You look like you're . . . getting better."

They were lying. This is what The Kidney Makeover did to my body: My legs turned into tree trunks. When I walked, my blubbery thighs slapping together sounded like elephants humping. My face ballooned up until it was a perfectly round moon. My signature skinny arms still looked like dental floss, but my stomach was so rock-hard, distended, and swollen, that I was this close to applying for a Pea in the Pod credit card. I had nightmares about my boss asking me to strap my new man-breasts down with a size 38DDD bra.

The Kidney Makeover did have its upside. I'd always had this thin horselike face and suddenly I had big fat rosy cheeks, like a Gerber Baby. And I finally had a derriere, for the first time in my life. I wasn't born with a butt. I'd thought about buying one on the Internet at buyabutt.com, but I could only afford one synthetic cheek—and now, suddenly, I had back. It was a juicy, protruding, hot, fat, meaty, no-messing-around caboose. I was so proud of my multilevel, walks-into-the-room-and-gets-wedged-in-a-doorway, heaping kiss-my-ass buns. I will tell you all a secret: When I was taking my post-surgery walks around Cedars-Sinai I would keep my hospital gown untied just so I could show off that boot. I suddenly understood what it was like to be Beyoncé.

Seriously, though, the weight issue hit close to home: I have a long hidden history of weight struggles. If my body issues were a Montel episode, it would be titled "I Was A Teenage Manorexic." When I was sixteen, I thought I had to look like Iggy Pop. I knew I was never going to look like a blonde-haired, blue-eyed, golden-boy jock with a jawline of steel. But a quirky, emaciated rock star? That I could do. I had already been ostracized for being the school freak. I wasn't allowed anywhere near the popular circles. The Goths were willing to take me in, as long as I went on the Goth Starvation Diet. To be a Goth you had to have a 26-inch waistline.

So I stopped eating. My one meal of the day, eaten at lunchtime, would be a piece of melba toast and a sliver of mozzarella cheese. And that was it. All of the sudden I went from being powerless to feeling powerful. Every day, I climbed on the scale and watched my weight drop. It was absolute control. It became a really sick game: I would delight in how long I could go without food. Hunger was the enemy, and I scoffed at it. Hunger was no match for me. What a triumph.

I started the beginning of my junior year weighing a healthy 160 pounds. Nine months later, I weighed 132 pounds (on a 6-foot frame) and had become the scandal of my community. I was the walking dead.

There were epic battles with my parents. My father would try to physically terrorize me into sitting down for dinner. My mother would just weep. When they forced me to eat, I started taking laxatives, and then vomiting. My mother could hear me gagging in the bathroom after meals, so I would turn the tap on to mask the sound. I thought that my contribution to the world would be a technique to vomit silently.

But the community was speaking, and once I was the buzz of the town, it was all over. We never went to a professional, because in a dysfunctional Canadian-Romanian Jewish family, you don't go outside for help; but somehow—with bullying and tough love—my parents eventually made me eat.

Not long after I was diagnosed with PKD, I suddenly recalled my teenage struggle with manorexia. It was like a knife went through me; I got goose bumps all over. I thought, *Maybe this is a result of when I had food issues when I was sixteen, and took all those laxatives.*

OH NO! IT'S MY FAULT. I was panicked at the idea that I had done this—all the suffering, everything that I was going to lose—by my own hand, because I had been a fool as a teenager and didn't eat for nine months. I lacerated myself, tore myself apart for being so stupid.

Eventually, my doctor told me that I was being irrational. "It's genetic," he said. "You didn't bring this on yourself." PKD was in my blood all along, along with the gene for thick luxurious hair.

My parents, however, refused to believe this. "How did you get it?" my mother asked.

"It's genetic," I said. "I got it from one of you."

"Nononononono," my mother said. "Not my side of the family. It's impossible." She looked at my father, instead. My mother has always romanticized the notion that she married way beneath her; so of course PKD must have come from his peasant genes, his plebeian blood.

My father backpedaled. "Nononononono, it's not *my* family, Amelia! It's from *your* side."

"Nononononononono!" I left them there to bicker. I think my father slept on the faux-Oriental divan for at least two weeks.

As an adult, I had given up on the laxatives and melba toast, but I was still obsessed with my weight. In the years before I was diagnosed with PKD, I was fanatically concerned with fitting into body-hugging clothes. There's a sickness in high fashion: Stars starve themselves to fit into size zero samples, and men's clothes are cut for six-foot tall Nordic models who are nineteen years old with miracle metabolisms.

At my skinniest on the red carpet, I weighed 145 pounds. I

thought I looked like the spawn of Mick Jagger. But really I was the walking near-dead. There's a photograph of me from the Oscars in 2004, before I got ill that I've looked at a lot lately. I'm wearing a silver satin tux, and I look so hollow and sickly. It made me see how twisted my perception of myself had been for the longest time.

Now, after all those years of being ultra-thin and wearing anything I wanted, the karmic fashion police had finally come around to get me for back payment. Now that I was taking steroids and doing dialysis, my skinny designer clothes had gotten so tight that I thought they would have to be donated to the Fashion Critics Hall of Fame. I could hardly breathe in them. But I still tried to wear them anyway. I thought the tighter my pants were, the more the fat would be compressed. It didn't work. In one last attempt at vanity, I finally reached into the back of my closet, unlocked the safe, and pulled out the ultimate emergency fat-busting weapon in my arsenal: A girdle. Wearing a discreet Ralph Lauren pith helmet and a to-die-for khaki jungle suit, I had slipped unnoticed into the Macy's women's undergarment department. I was dizzy with confusion as I tried to decipher the differences between a Nancy Ganz Hip Slip and a Spanx Power Panty.

An older woman in cat glasses and a red beehive came up behind me. "Ahem," she cleared her throat. "Can I help you?"

"I have an ailing aunt. It's her eightieth birthday and the retirement home is throwing a dance party. And between you and me, hon, her belly is the size of the Domican Republic."

"Oh dollface," she said. "Thank God you've come to Irma. What she needs is the Turbo-Charged Ionic Belly Vise. Trust me, she'll look like Petra Nemcova."

I wore that Belly Vise underneath my white evening jacket and black tux pants at the Emmys soon after. Irma was wrong. I was not as lithe as Petra Nemcova. Not only were my air vents so constricted that I almost fainted into Kiefer Sutherland's arms, I still looked like my own gated community.

At home, when I was by myself, I would disrobe and look in the mirror from every angle. I spent hours in the bathroom, just gazing at my grotesque form. I was losing the battle of the bulge. I had a primal fear that this was something I was going to have to come to terms with: I was terrified that I would never be slender again. As my stomach continued to swell, day after day, I started having panic attacks that I would never see my privates again—at least, not without a hand mirror.

My response: It wasn't eating a healthy diet or exercising more. No, instead, I discovered sugar. In the dark days after losing the kidney and going on dialysis, sugar was the only thing I had in my life that was making me happy. It filled some sort of void. It became my crutch.

I would make trips to my local over-priced coffee emporium to get the triple grande sugar heroin-in-a-cup surprise delight with whipped cream. I'd have about three a day. I'd eat boxes of designer chocolates, cartons of milk chocolate truffles, buckets of ice cream. Even my food-obsessed mother grew concerned when she came to visit. "You have to stop," she would tell me, although that didn't mean that she stopped baking me the cupcakes that I craved.

Sugar was my form of rebellion against a life full of restrictions. I'm a man who hates rules, and here I was in a medical prison, forbidden to drink alcohol and smoke cigarettes. My schedule was filled with pills and machines. Enter the sugar: The chocolate rushes became my way of acting out. I can speak from experience that a box of Godiva was more powerful than a morphine drip and 30 Vicodin mixed into a latte. It sent my whole body into overdrive with sugar tremors.

I knew that sugar was bad for my physical and mental health. I was already about to explode from the drugs and dialysis and weight gain; by adding sugar addiction to steroids I was entering dangerous territory.

The tipping point came when I was searching for clothes for another awards show and realized that I had become a second-class citizen. I went to stores and felt invisible: "We don't carry higher than size 44," the salespeople would tell me. "Our clothes aren't cut for your type of body," they would sniff. Luckily I had padding, because I practically fell on my ass with shock.

I felt discriminated against and victimized. I'd never been so humiliated in my life. It shook me up. Initially, I was fixated on the number: I had to be a size 40 suit again. But eventually I realized I was thinking about losing weight for the wrong reasons. It made me take a long hard look at myself and realize that I had to lose weight because I felt bad, physically. I was dragging, easily out of breath and my doctor said that with my condition, I was more prone to diabetes.

I didn't go on a special diet: Dr. Jordan just said, "You need a sensible, heart-healthy plan." For him, that meant lean meats and vegetables, watch the salt and sugar, and get lots of exercise. I signed up with a personal trainer, who tortured me with exercise balls and push-ups ad nauseum three times a week. Since I have a Cleopatra complex and believe that I should have everything delivered to me, I signed up for an organic food service to bring me my meals. I cut out wheat and dairy almost entirely.

I never dreamed I'd be thin again. I thought that was too much to ask for. But after a year of dieting, giving up sodium and sweets and late-night snacks, eating organic woodchips and alfalfa sprouts for dinner, exercising and power-walking two miles a day, I knocked off a considerable amount of weight. For the first time in my life, I lost weight the sane way—and it stuck.

But it was a bitter victory, because when I lost the weight my butt also took off without even leaving a Dear John letter. Once again, I was buttless. Bye-bye backside.

CHAPTER 12

Mr. Bloated Red Carpet Fancy Pants

It's the end of August, and I am relaxing at P. Diddy's dinner party at the Setai Hotel in South Beach, Miami, before the MTV VMA awards. The lobby has been transformed into a chic Zen den—it's very Polynesian monastary. I think I'm leaning on a mahogany column when it suddenly moves, and says, "Hey sexy": The pole is actually Paris Hilton, who appears to be suffering from an advanced case of pre-melanoma spray-tan poisoning.

I am wearing a white suit with a fuschia shirt and a white se-quinned tie. This outfit was supposed to show people that Cojo Is Back! But it's a lie. I'm still a complete mess. I believe that white is always the freshest and most glamorous color choice, but I'm forty pounds overweight and feel almost as big as the Gulfstream GV that flew Diddy into town.

I'm bloated beyond recognition from steroids. On my way to pay my respects to P. Diddy, I'm worried that I'll have to hand over my dental records for him to recognize me, but even through the folds of flesh and the pudgy face he remembers who I am: "How you doing, Cojo? Good to see you!" he says.

I slip out early, before midnight, when the party is still just getting started, and head back to my hotel room. I take off the white suit and the fuschia shirt, exposing the tube that has been sewn into my stomach, and put on rubber gloves and a face mask. And then I start setting up my dialysis machine. There are sealed bags of solution that need to be opened in a particular way, sterilized to prevent infection, and warmed so that the cold fluids won't shock my system. Three IV drips have to be set up—two for the dextrose compound that will go into my stomach and another for the waste that will come out. New tubing has to be sterilized and attached to my stomach. My beautiful room at the Ritz is piled high with boxes and bags of fluid.

The peritoneal dialysis machine sits on the nightstand. I turn it on, plug myself in, climb into my bed and then drift off to sleep. In the lobby of the Setai, P. Diddy is still swigging Cristal with Pharrell. But there will be no bubbly for me tonight. Instead, for the next nine hours, my body will alternately be pumped full of chemicals and then drained like a sewer.

Competitive me, I had attended peritoneal dialysis school all through July with a vengeance, determined to be my instructor Doris's star pupil. Doris was my drill sergeant: A curmudgeon with a heaving breast and a personality of steel. Underneath, she was all warmth, but I've never been more afraid of someone in my life. "Peritonitis is our enemy!" she would trill, as she hovered over me and watched me struggle with the tubes.

In high school, I wasn't exactly an A student. I would skip class to go to Brown's Shoes in Cavendish Mall; I'd visit the men's section and just subtly, accidentally . . . my goodness, how did I find myself in the women's section looking at all the strappy stilettos? But this was not like that. Whatever gray matter I had was devoted fully to the process of learning peritoneal dialysis: This was life or death, and it required 1,000 percent laserlike focus. I was going to be Phi Beta Kappa Kappa Kappa—the ultimate graduate—or nothing at all.

I've always been the Sultan of Squeamish. I would hold my tinkle on an airplane for five hours rather than brave the horrors of an airplane lavatory. When I got my ear pierced, I lost my lunch. But I was getting over it, big time. When you have no choice but to fight for your life, and that's simply the cards that have been dealt to you, you *have* to get over it.

Still, the first few times I tried peritoneal by myself, I was terrified: I had my life in my own hands. And I was bad at it—I kept screwing up. Doris's instructions came in a cheap plastic blue binder, which was my bible: There were thirty steps in it, printed up on color-coded laminated sheets. Important steps were in blazing red—sterilizing the end of the tube that had been sewn into my stomach, removing any air bubbles that might have compromised the dextrose cleaning solution. There were bags and tubes everywhere, and I had to be meticulous about making sure the right tube ended up in the right solution. If I did anything wrong, an alarm would go off and the machine would flash warning instructions. Panicked, I would call Doris for help, even if it was three o'clock in the morning.

By mid-August, six weeks after my infected kidney had been removed, I had been doing peritoneal dialysis at home for a month. I still felt overwhelmed and petrified every single minute I was on it, but I was starting to live my life again, slowly. I would go to the *Entertainment Tonight* stage to work. I went back on the Beverly Hills ladies-who-lunch circuit, where I would arrive with freshly done hair and impeccable nails, and could always be counted on to deliver the latest dish. But my disease refused to leave me alone.

One afternoon, I was clinking crystal glasses with society swells over endive salad at a Diane Von Furstenberg lunch, flushed with happiness that I was out again, a thousand light-years away from the disease, but afterward, after waiting by the valet stand in the blazing sun for twenty minutes, *I fainted* from heat, exhaustion, and dehydration. A size–0 society matron in a printed wrap dress that matched her liver spots somehow managed to throw me over her shoulder and carry me inside the cool shop.

Despite such minor humiliations, I insisted on getting back out in the social scene. I *wasn't* the same person anymore. I was weak. I was *straining* to be the life of the party, like I didn't have a care in the world. I wanted so badly to appear normal, so that no one would treat me differently. I had too much pride to be thought of as sick. So no one heard about my nightly dialysis procedures. No one had to hear about the pain I still dealt with, or the indescribable aches, or the fainting spells, or the dehydration.

I love being a crybaby. Give me any chance to whine and complain, and I'll take it. As the former captain of the Beverly Hills Whining Squad, I thought that with kidney disease, at least it would give me a license to whine away. But the ghost of Jackie O texted and the message said, "Steven, decorum is everything. Silence is the most noble thing."

Instead, I would be at some chic dinner party yakking away with Kirsten Dunst and sharing lemon-hummus dip with Penelope Cruz. And then I would come home and be slapped once again in the face with reality: Even though I just wanted to moisturize and fall into bed, I had to spend half an hour sterilizing and heating and setting up tubes. Would it go smoothly that night? Would the machine alarm go off? My nights always ended with fear.

Still, despite the tenuous nature of my life, I was crawling out of my skin to get out on the red carpet again. I wasn't ready, physically *or* emotionally, but I felt like my career would be over if I didn't. I hadn't worked on the red carpet in almost a year; the closest I'd been was my remote Oscar appearance eight months earlier. It felt like I'd been gone for a millennium.

I felt that I had something to prove—to the world, and to myself. So at the end of August I decided to go on the Dialysis Tour. Stop one: the VMAs in Miami. Stop two: New York, to do a special for *The Insider*. Stop three: The Emmys in Los Angeles. Stop four: Chicago, for a follow-up appearance on *Oprah*. As always, I would be traveling with my pooch, my BlackBerry, a beauty supply store on wheels, and my camera crew. But this time, I would be bringing along a new assistant: My dialysis machine.

Hurricanes swept through Miami a few days before I got on a plane to go to the VMAs. They nearly cancelled the party. I called Shari in a panic: "What if there is a power failure because of the hurricane and I can't plug my dialysis machine in? What if I get stranded in the middle of nowhere without my dialysis machine? If I miss even one day, the doctor says the toxins will build up in my body and make me sick. Should I even go?"

Shari told me I was making a mistake. "Put your health first!" She warned me. But I didn't listen. I wanted to be busy and stimulated and occupied by the things I knew. I wanted to see celebrities in ill-fitting dresses and with botched boob jobs, leaking saline all over the red carpet.

I brought my dialysis machine on board the airplane with me, in a special wheeled carrier bag, along with a note from Doris explaining to security that I was a transplantee traveling with life-sustaining medical equipment. The actual bags of dialysis solution were supposed to be shipped to my hotel, but I couldn't help thinking, *What if the boxes don't arrive at all? What will I do?*

I carried my drugs with me in a plastic ziplock freezer bag. My entire clock was still set around when I had to take my pills, forty of them a day. There were syrups, powders to be mixed with water, ghastly tasting liquids that I took with a spoon. It was ironic: I hadn't even been allowed to take aspirin as a child and now I'd become a walking pharmacy. Before, I could barely swallow a pill; now I felt like the Jenna Jameson of pill takers, deep-throating thirty pills in one gulp.

On the plane to Miami, I nearly gnawed apart the airplane safety card with anxiety. Fortunately, when I arrived at my hotel, I greeted the safely delivered boxes of dialysis equipment with the same glee that I once greeted bags of free premiere swag.

When my wake-up call rang the following morning, I got my real wake-up call: My posh hotel room had been transformed into a makeshift dialysis center, with syringes and pills bottles everywhere. The maid probably thought it was a travelling meth lab. I unplugged myself from the machine, emptied three bags of body waste down the drain of the beautiful marble tub. When I finished I took a shower, did a nutrient caviar hair mask, and let hair and makeup transform me into Mr. Red Carpet Fancy Pants. I was worried about being back on the red carpet, for the first time in almost a year. Would I be able to do my job after such a scarring, intense experience? Did I still have the same Chatty Cathy Cojo in me?

But it doesn't take a lot of sense memory to dive back into philosophical discourse with Jessica Simpson about lip waxing. It wasn't like I was leading a scientific inquiry into drug trials for parasitic infections. The truth was I slipped back into fluffdom so easily that it was alarming to me: I went from emergency rooms and hospitals and biopsies to speaking pig latin with Shakira in the blink of an eye. It kind of scared me how ingrained the superficial Hollywood bon vivant in me really was.

The stars were incredibly polite. Not one person mentioned my size—which was pretty generous, considering that I've eviscerated half of Hollywood. Instead, most of them showed genuine concern for my situation, even interrupting our interviews to quiz me: "How are you feeling? I'm glad you're well!"

I was growing comfortable with being the Prince of PKD. Sure, I was weak and disoriented, and my feet weren't quite on the ground. But even though I had been on a sabbatical, I still felt a part of it. I knew all the players on that carpet.

There was Gwyneth, walking down the red carpet, a breath of fresh air: Her husband, Chris Martin of Coldplay, was performing at the ceremony. Gwyneth had just had a baby and her lactating breasts were spilling out her top. She lit up when she saw me and pulled me aside to murmur in my ear. "Coj," she whispered urgently. "You have to tell me: Are my boobs everywhere?" she asked.

Somewhere in her cleavage, I staked a flag. Cojo had landed.

Kidney etiquette is very clear. You do not flat out ask someone to give you a kidney. You can't put them on the spot like that. Instead, you just have to hope that people will come forward and offer. You *do* sigh a lot on the telephone and say, "Pardon me, my dialysis machine has just lost power and I'm going to die in fourteen minutes if I don't get a kidney." But you try to be subtle about it.

After I lost Abby's kidney, I called in a repairman to oil the hinges on my front door because I was waiting for the stampede of friends and family who would be breaking it down to offer me a kidney. I needn't have worried about the door. People changed the subject, avoided the topic, danced around an offer. Perhaps out of guilt they would say "I'd love to give you a kidney, but . . ." There was always a but. I couldn't blame them. They had families, boyfriends and girlfriends, children.

By September of 2005 I was starting to feel desperate. I had heard whispers from other patients that it was possible to go to a foreign country and buy an organ. I was told that Southeastern Europe and Southwestern Asia were the It spots for kidneys, the Turks and Caicos of the organ trade, where you could pick up a fresh kidney for the American markup rate of $100,000. I entertained the idea for a second, but I quickly pulled myself back from the brink. As Dr. Jordan put it, "You're at an amazing American facility and you already lost a kidney. What would happen in a place with less than optimal care?" The risks were high, and I couldn't live with myself knowing the moral questions involved. Who knew where that kidney came from, or how its owner parted with it?

Meanwhile, I was starting to get kidney offers from a place I hadn't expected: People who had heard about my plight on *ET* or *The Insider* or *Oprah*. My inbox was full of notes from strangers who were offering to give me their internal organs, and I was shocked to be the recipient of such widespread, self-sacrificing generosity.

If you need a kidney, I'm here. That is, of course, if you don't mind having a woman, a Jewban (I'm Cuban and Jewish), filtering for you. My offer comes from the heart. Besides, I have two kidneys, and I was in school the day they taught sharing!!

Dear Cojo, I hope you don't think that I'm a crazed fan. I am listed as an organ donor if something were to happen to me, but I would also like to be tested for you as well. I think you are great, and it hurts me to see you like you are.

Hey Cojo. I'll give you a kidney, you gimme a makeover. I think that's pretty fair, huh?

The kidney offers from viewers touched me more than anything will ever touch me in my life. My friends began to set up a screening process, making phone calls to interview the people who had made serious offers. But just when we were starting to pursue this as a viable option, Dr. Jordan called me with an unexpected proposition: "I think we should talk about testing your mother."

I had never seriously considered this as a possibility until Dr.

Jordan had uttered her name. My family had held a mandatory town hall Cojocaru conference when I lost Abby's kidney: Both my sister and my father wanted to give me their kidneys, but neither turned out to be a match. The only family member I refused to consider was my mother: I had her on a pedestal—she was precious cargo, fine and delicate, and 70 years old. I would call 911 if she got a mole. I was never going to consider putting her in any danger.

So when Dr. Jordan suggested testing her, I stopped breathing for a second and almost blacked out. My first thought was, *What?! You want to kill my mother? You want to put my mother on the operating table and scoop a kidney out of her?* It was one of the only times in my life that I was speechless—save for being on the operating table myself.

"What are you talking about?" I finally stammered. "Where is this coming from?"

"I've known your mother for a while now," Dr. Jordan said. "She is an incredibly spry, robust, healthy woman for her age. She looks and acts like she's much younger than she really is. We should test her. Maybe she's an option."

In the kidney community, doctors talk a lot about the perfect kidney candidate. It's a morbid discussion. They talk about the allegorical, metaphorical football player who is twenty years old, strong, the picture of health, with a vital, active, dynamic fresh kidney. But in order for that kidney to be available for a transplant, the football player has to have one final touchdown—literally.

My mother was the antithesis of that football player. But she had the potential to be a much better match for me than any quarterback. "You would need fewer drugs, because she would be a genetic match," Dr. Jordan explained.

"Isn't she ancient?" I asked.

"It's been done before with family members who are that age," he said. "Just let me test her for blood typing, and then we can talk."

That week, my mother was visiting from Montreal. When I told her that Dr. Jordan had recommended that we test her, she started dancing around the house. I'd never seen her that happy—well, maybe at my bar mitzvah after two rum & cokes. She was so giddy that her voice went up fifteen octaves. "I am giving you a kidney!" she yelled.

"No, don't be ridiculous. We're just talking about it as a maybe-maybe, probably not a real option," I told her. I thought that this was something serious that we would discuss and deliberate about. My mother had no intention of the sort.

"No," she replied. "I feel it in my bones I am going to give you a kidney."

She left for Montreal a few days later, gave blood at a hospital there, and within weeks we had determined that she was a match. It presented me with the ultimate moral dilemma. I wanted her kidney. I did. But I also didn't. The natural instinct for self-preservation and survival was clashing with the other natural instinct of putting your loved ones before you. No wonder I was so torn up inside. I was deathly afraid for my mother.

Inside, I was also feeling guilty for even thinking about using her kidney to pull myself out of my hooked-up-to-a-machine hell. Secretly, I wanted my new kidney to come from my mother: We were the same person, it was meant to be. In the end, I knew that her kidney would be my salvation. But even for me, the most self-absorbed narcissist on the planet, this felt like a new world record of selfishness.

By the time October rolled around, my mother had been poked, prodded, tested, and retested. The doctors examined every organ twice, gave her blood tests, stress tests, psychological tests, heart tests. She had to see a dozen different doctors. She was a total trooper, never complaining, never once showing any fear. *I* was the one who spent my days on pins and needles.

Rather than making a decision one way or another, I was a wimp: I let events unfold without my input. A committee at Cedars-Sinai convened to discuss my mother's kidney candidacy and came back with a unanimous verdict: It would be safe to use her as a donor.

"She is the perfect candidate for you," Dr. Jordan told me. "It couldn't be a better match. And she's in such great shape that I really don't think it's a big risk."

So I added yet another surgery to my datebook: On October 11, 2005, my mother would be giving me her kidney.

CHAPTER 14

One Tarnished Belly Ring, Manischewitz
Wine Spritzers, and Air Kisses from the Gurney

My personal emergency hotline when I'm in an emotional maelstrom is 1–800-SHARI. The Cojo Clan had swooped down on my tranquil abode with all their bombastic love and familiar dysfunction. My mother was about to go under the knife and, two for the price of one, so was I. I was thinking the unthinkable: Would Mom survive the operation? And what was my kidney transplant sequel going to be: Box office bonanza? Or an opening weekend flop, where the kidney never takes?

I was getting an ulcer worrying about surviving: Not just the surgery, but surviving my high-strung, overwrought family and their theatrics. Who else would I reach out to—who could orchestrate her way through this madness and hold my delicate paw—but Shari, the childhood friend who loved me even when I had a unibrow and buck teeth? I put her in charge of directing all the emotional traffic.

Shari flew in the day before the surgery. When I picked her up at the airport, I didn't mince words about what I needed. "My father and sister are freaking out since half the family is about to be filleted at Cedars tomorrow morning," I told her. "I need a break from all this tension. My sister keeps looking at me like I'm a mother murderer, and my father has dueling rabbis saying prayers, one for me and one for Mom."

"OK," Shari said. "Let's have a live-for-the-moment day. Let's run away."

Her words gave me the strength to do cartwheels: "Let's run away" are my three favorite words, in Latin, English, or Swahili.

The spiritual journey began at Fred Segal in Santa Monica. Shari announced that it was time to get a new hospital look, and she was buying.

"Well, since you put it that way," I said. "I'm feeling *fresh*. Renewed. This transplant is a new beginning: I need the sartorial equivalent of a Summer's Eve douche."

We immediately conference-called Zac Posen to consult on a fabulous new direction for my hospital wardrobe. "Cashmere is so two minutes ago," he declared. "I think luxurious smooth cottons are mad-chic. Think crisp. Think St. Barts."

"Yes, yes, Zac!" I cried. "I see me in cotton palazzos and a lighter-than-air chemise, very Nautica model meets Portofino gigolo!"

Shari shrieked at the entire Fred Segal's salestaff. "Get me every single piece of cotton you have in the store. And give me colors! I want primrose! Seafoam! Coral!"

From there, we cruised to Malibu, a place where it feels like disease doesn't exist. We drove with the top down, caution to the wind, bombing down the freeway as we broke the barriers of sound and light. We giggled as we looked at our wind-whipped tumbleweed 'dos. Shari had brought her 1970s supermixes with her—the kind of music that worms its way into your brain and gives you an embolism—and demanded that we play "Shake Your Groove Thing" on an endless loop.

It was sensory overload: The gorgeous white sand beaches, the waves on the coastline, the seagulls swooping overhead. Shari was humming along off-tune, beating the dashboard. We stopped at a liquor store and bought Peach Nectar wine coolers and guzzled them out of brown paper bags. Hammered, Shari shook her hair out and began wolf-whistling the surfers that we drove by: "Nice butt, beach boy!" I ripped off my shirt, slathered my chest in baby oil, revved up my motor and challenged a Subaru Outback to a drag race.

The end of the day found us passed out on the beach, my chest burnt to crimson, the empty baby oil bottles tossed in a heap nearby, Shari's sexy 'do a rats-nest of sand, sweat, and sea kelp. The Peach Nectar buzz had worn off.

I looked at Shari, facedown in the sand, and something came over me. I was warmed by the knowledge that I had such a solid friend, a partner in crime, an ally in my kidney war. I began to think of the transplant the next morning, of my mother undergoing surgery, of the long recovery I still faced after my transplant. My first transplant had initially felt like a fairy tale: Going in, I didn't really believe that anything could go wrong with that kidney. But this time I knew the reality of my situation, all the different things that could happen, and I didn't like the odds.

Shari noticed that my face had changed. "What are you thinking?" she asked.

"Shari, am I doing the right thing by putting my mom through this?" I said. "Tell me the truth. I can't think straight anymore. Tell me what to do."

"Everything will be OK," she said. "Your mom is going to be fine. You have doctors who have been very positive about this surgery."

I was still quiet: "I feel so selfish taking a kidney from my mother," I said.

Shari shook her head. "It's not being selfish," she said. "Look: I've talked to your mother, and she wants to give you this kidney with all her heart: She's doing it with so much love. Even if she has to hit you over the head until you're unconscious, she's giving you this kidney. She feels like it's her purpose, to save your life.

"This has brought her the first joy she's had since you were diagnosed last year," she continued. "You have to understand that. She's giving you a gift, and you have to take it. It's not being selfish. So stop worrying: We'll get through this. It's all going to be good."

One side effect of my disease was that, after more than a year of struggle, I was finally starting to listen to people in a way I never had before. I was learning to trust: People like Dr. Jordan. Dr. Cohen, Doris the Dialysis Diva, even my parents. I *wasn't* in control; everything *wasn't* in my hands; and I needed to trust the people around me who were telling me what to do. At that moment, I trusted Shari, my personal social worker. Listening to her words, I decided to stop worrying, as much as I could. My whole family was coming together to face the biggest challenge of our lives. I needed them, and they needed me.

No medical procedure in my life—whether it be a reverse vasectomy or a mole removal—is complete without a television camera nearby to record it. *Entertainment Tonight* was taping the preparations for my second transplant and, the night before the surgery, they arrived to capture what was supposed to be the perfect nuclear family enjoying a lovely home-cooked meal the evening before this big milestone. It was a coming-together-in-crisis repast. I was envisioning a soothing evening together, just me, my family, Shari, and half a dozen members of the film crew.

I called my mother on the way home from Malibu to check in on the dinner preparations. While Shari and I were on the beach, my parents had been cooking: They were the poor man's Mario Batali and Paula Deen, dancing around the kitchen together as they sprinkled bread crumbs over everything in sight.

"Is everything ready for *ET*?" I asked.

"Darling. Everything is perfect, it's *gorjus*. I made your favorite, triple-layer lasagna and roast chicken, so gorjus. It's melt in your mouth!" she gushed. In the background, I could hear my father singing "That's Amore." "We have the candles, and I brought Grandma's crocheted tablecloth!"

"What's Alisa doing?" I asked. "Did she help you?"

"You must be joking. Your sister is on the terrace, getting a tan."

I arrived home feeling very Zen after my fantasy day with Shari, oozing good energy as I floated toward the front door. As we were about to walk in, Shari whispered one final time: "Don't let anyone get to you," she said. "Let's enjoy this dinner."

"Of course," I said. My promise lasted about a nanosecond.

My parents flung open the front door with cries of delight, hugs and kisses all around. And then my sister came leaping into the living room to say hello.

I adore Alisa, but her wardrobe has always been a bone of contention. She may be a woman of a certain age, not far off from a hot flash, but she dresses like Hannah Montana. She is adorable, only five feet tall, 105 pounds (97 without makeup and accessories), with the body of an eighteen-year-old and those gorgeous Cojocaru legs. But I'm mortified by her skintight skirts, her platform heels, the glitter tube tops that she wears to synagogue.

That day, she was prepped and ready for the *ET* camera crews in a day-glo orange cut-off midriff tank top, spray-on jeans, and four inch-high Lucite wedges. Her shimmering, shiny, sunken stomach was doused with sparkling body lotion. My eyes went straight to her belly button. And there! Could it be? Was it? Incredulous, I looked closer. It was the darkest moment in the history of the Cojocaru family: My sister was wearing a belly ring in public.

"What are you wearing!" I shrieked. "Are you insane?"

"What?" Alisa bleated. She looked down at her belly button. "What's wrong with this?"

"You are four hundred twenty years old and you are wearing a *belly ring?* Do you think you are Janet Jackson? You are a plague on this family! A social embarassment! You need electroshock therapy!"

WWIII had erupted. My dad began to scream at Alisa: "You see? I told you so. How many times have I told you to stop dressing like that? You should be ashamed of yourself."

My sister had tears in her eyes. "What's wrong? This is California! This outfit is *normal*!"

Shari had fled. Stinky ducked for cover under the couch. The dogs in the neighborhood were howling in response to the frequency of my shrieks. I fished out my wallet, took out a fifty dollar bill, and threw it at Alisa. "Go stay at the stripper hotel down the street with all the other pole dancers. You're not staying here looking like that!"

The pent-up stress inside me had finally found its outlet. I could have talked until I was blue in the face about being rational, visited a dozen therapists, taken three different antidepressants, but the truth was that I was an emotional wreck, and the one person guaranteed to set me off was my sister. It was full-scale blitzkrieg.

Alisa ran away, as fast as you can run in platform heels. In the kitchen, my dad clanged pots furiously. My mother fretted in the living room. Doors slammed all over the house. Finally, my sister emerged upstairs in a virgin-white Donna Karan cashmere sweater set.

"Thank God," I said. The Cojos move on very quickly: By the time the *ET* crews arrived, everything was back to normal again. Soon, my sister was laughing so hard that the Manischewitz wine was coming out of her nose. My dad was eating his third helping of lasagna. And I was regaling the family with X-rated stories about the Olsen twins. We forgot that anything had happened at all and that anything out of the ordinary was going to happen the following day either.

Still, before I went to bed that night, I gave my sister a list of everything she was forbidden to wear to the hospital: Sheer tops. Fishnets of any kind. Rubber. Anything that lit up on the nipples.

T-shirts with bull's-eyes on them, or anything that said "Honk if you like my puppies."

The next morning at Cedars-Sinai, my mother was practically beating down the door to get into surgery: She was practically jumping out of her skin. She paced back and forth, pleading with the nurses, "Take me! Take me now! I can't wait another second to give my son my kidney!"

When the nurses did come to take to her to pre-op, there was no time for a big dramatic emotional moment. I wanted to clutch at her, but she was consumed by her rush to get to the operating room. I was blubbering. I was mush. But my mom was noble: Her head was high and she was peaceful and gracious and proud. She touched my cheeks and held me without saying anything.

Before she left, she whispered in my ear, "I can't wait to wake up and know that you are well."

As the rest of the family sat waiting in Robin's office for the moment when I'd be carted away to the operating room again, it was my sister who cried the most. I was headed into surgery, my father was silently watching his wife and his son go under the knife, Shari was holding my hand so tightly that it was about to snap off, but it was my sister who was the most distraught, and I loved her for it.

As I was finally wheeled off to the operating room, I made a mock-sour face at Alisa: Here we go. I blew her a kiss from the gurney, and we both smiled. Blood is blood.

CHAPTER 15

El Cojo Puede Hacer Pis
(or The Tinkle Heard Around the World)

My eyes blearily cracked open. My head was throbbing. My heavy eyes were like little slits, and I could barely make out my surroundings. I began to cough in a way I'd never coughed before: I couldn't catch my breath. What was going on with my throat? What was going on with my *mouth*? My tongue was pressed against a cold plastic object: Something was lodged in my throat.

I had some kind of breathing tube in my mouth! I started to gag. Where was I? I opened my eyes wider and tried desperately to focus.

This wasn't a hospital room: I was in some kind of a holding tank, an empty windowless space with a lot of growling machines. I was completely alone. I wanted to reach up and rip the tube out of my mouth, but I couldn't move my arm. It was strapped down. *I* was strapped down.

Every movement was a struggle, but the adrenaline was driving me: I kicked and heaved violently, like a trapped animal, trying to break free. I felt like I was drowning, submerged, claustrophobic: I wanted desperately to breathe on my own.

It was like being in a mental ward, and I thought I was losing my mind. Disoriented, I didn't know what had happened to me: How long had I been under? Was it a day later or a year? I felt as if I'd woken up into an Edgar Allan Poe story, the one where the protagonist is buried alive. Maybe I *had* been buried alive. Maybe I was *dead*. Hearing my struggle, a nurse ran into the room and quickly stabbed me with a needle. "You are in the ICU, on a ventilator," he told me. "You have to calm down. Everything is OK."

"Take it out!" I tried to scream. The only sound that came out of my mouth was a gurgling moan. But the sedative was working and within seconds I had been sent back into oblivion.

I woke up again hours later to see my father hovering over the bed. It took me a moment to focus. The ventilator was gone, but my throat still ached.

"Dad, what happened? What's going on?" I asked him. My voice was dry and scratchy.

"There was a problem," he told me. "Just after the transplant operation, when you were still in the recovery room, an alarm went off. Something went wrong with the arteries in your legs, and they had to operate on you again. Your kidney, to protect itself, has shut itself down. But they say it will wake up."

I wanted to cry. The kidney wasn't working? I thought I'd earned so much karma over the last year that it was time for a payback.

"How is Mom?" I asked, afraid to even hear. "Is she OK?"

"Your mom is terrific, everything is fine with her," he said. His voice cracked as he looked at me. "Your sister and I were pacing the hallways."

My father and I have clashed over our lifetime: probably because I would walk right over him to get to my mother. But at that moment it was just me and him. "Steven, I'm so proud of you," he said. "You have been so great. We are all together in this." It was the validating moment that every boy dreams off: The big father-son moment, as real and raw as you can get.

"I love you, Dad," I said. "Thank you so much for everything you've done for me."

A few minutes later, Dr. Cohen came in to explain the situation. The new kidney wasn't dead, he promised. After the transplant, I had what they called a "vascular complication," and the blood stopped flowing in my legs. Dr. Cohen had to operate immediately in order to open up my circulation again. My clever kidney had simply gone to sleep to protect itself from the shock. "I have seen this a thousand times," Dr. Cohen told me. "I know it well. It might take a few weeks for your kidney to wake up."

"Is there a chance it *won't* wake up?" I asked. "Because I don't think I can handle that, Dr. Cohen. Really. Just bring on the last, fatal dose of morphine if that's the case."

He shook his head. "No, this has happened with many of my patients. It *will* wake up. I'm not saying maybe, I'm saying it's just a matter of time. But we will have to put you back on dialysis . . ."

At that dreaded word I thought I might have to hit him over the head. I lost it completely. "No! No! I thought I was done with that? No way! You can't do this to me! Why is this happening?"

"Listen to Dr. Cohen," my father said, trying to quiet my hysteria. "The kidney is going to come back. It's just sleeping now."

"Well, tell it to *wake up*," I said. I didn't believe them. Inside, I was monumentally crushed. Here we were again: in a hospital room with a brand-new kidney that wasn't working. Once again, I had to fight to save an organ that someone I loved had given to me.

When my mother came down to visit me the next day, I tried to be upbeat. She had been recovering on the Club Floor, in the same Audrey Hepburn memorial suite that I'd recovered in, and had grown so beloved by the hospital staff that the nurses had taken to calling her "Mama." She was wheeled into the ICU looking pale and small, far from the dragonslayer I loved.

"Thank God it's over," I told her, trying to keep a smile on my face. "Thank you for saving me."

"I am the happiest mother in the world that I could do it," she smiled. "Happy is not even the big enough word."

I wished I could share her joy. I was back on dialysis; and when the doctors finally released me from the hospital, after nine days, the kidney still hadn't woken up. I was tortured by it. "It's going to come back," Doris, my dialysis instructor, promised me, as she sent me home with the peritoneal dialysis machine. "You'll see. Soon, you're going to start to urinate a lot. That will mean the kidney is alive and kicking."

It's easy to preach to sick people: "Be positive! It's all going to be all right!" But as much as positivity and faith had been the benchmarks of my story, it's not always possible to keep a smile on your face. Everyone around me was being a cheerleader, but I was in mourning. I was furious that this second transplant had been, in my mind, a disaster. I had been wronged by the world. This was my mother's sacred kidney! My mother = Mother Teresa! It didn't get more clear than that!

Returning home from Cedars-Sinai in late October was like experiencing déjà vu. I had another eight weeks of bedbound recovery in front of me, but this time with a kidney that still wasn't working and nightly dialysis sessions back on my calendar. I was once again on massive doses of steroids. My father was cooking up a storm. And my mother, despite her own pain, was playing Florence Nightingale: She baked cookies, coerced me to go on walks, made me watch *Sex and the City* at gunpoint. Forced cheeriness, like something from a Christmas television special, was the order of the day.

I just gave up and checked out. I had lost my mojo. I didn't want to leave my bed. Carrie Bradshaw wasn't doing it for me anymore. Even my mother's overwhelming optimism wouldn't lift me. The only thing that worked to dull my dismal mood was medication.

I had every drug at my disposal. For the most part, I had been careful not to indulge in them: At one point after losing the first kidney, I'd taken too much Vicodin, and Dr. Jordan had lectured me: "These drugs are not candy," he said. "They show up in your liver, and I can't have that. I need you healthy." I'd been a saint ever since. But now I wanted to stage a Feel Sorry For Myself Parade. My mother would come in to my room and beg me, "Come on, darling, let's walk upstairs for breakfast. Do it for me." I would gruffly tell her, no, not in the mood, and take a Valium. When that wore off, I'd take another tranquilizer. Maybe a Klonopin or two. A nice soothing Xanax. Or dip into the painkiller arsenal: Vicodin, Darvocet, and the real cherry on the cake, Percocet. I just wanted to flatline any emotion.

The days passed in a blur. It had already been ten days since my return home. During a commercial break of *Oprah* one afternoon, I crawled to the bathroom. As I stood, woozy, over the toilet, it came almost out of nowhere: I had struck oil. I was urinating like a Kauaian waterfall.

"Oh my God!" I screamed. "Mom! Mom! I can pee! I can pee! The kidney has woken up!"

From the bathroom, I could hear my mother's shrieks in the kitchen, and then footsteps scurrying down the stairs. Her purloined Peninsula Hotel houseslippers carried her to my bedroom door as fast as they would take her. "Is it true?" she asked.

I came out and flung my arms around her, even though she still had flour on her hands from making wienerschnitzel and fries. We jumped up and down and practically sang: "It's working! It's working!" I wanted the news flashing on JumboTron screens all over the world: COJO IS PEEING! I imagined people across the continents doing the wave in celebration, pictured the headlines of newspapers in fifty different languages: "El Cojo puede hacer pis!" "Le Cojo Urine!" "Cojo is naar de badkamers gegaan!"

In the days after it woke up, our little sleeping beauty was babied: My mother felt that if the kidney was nursed, carefully, it would thrive. We fed it my mother's secret cure-all puree of Matzoh ball soup, her melt-on-the-tongue beef brisket, and her twenty-four-hour-rise challah bread. She wanted to make sure the kidney had regular naps, daily walks, and plenty of sunlight: It got so ridiculous that I thought she would try to burp the kidney.

I decided not to give this kidney a name: everything had a different tenor this time around. I couldn't think of a better name than Mom's Kidney. Bathed in love, her kidney was humming along beautifully. In between naps, I would stroll over to the doctors for blood tests.

In late November, Jenny rang with an all-too-familiar story: "Your creatinine levels are up," she said. "We need to do a biopsy." I drove back to Cedars-Sinai with a sinking heart: *Was this kidney in danger, too? Was I repeating history?*

It was a false alarm, but it still left me unsettled. And just two weeks later, I hit another bump in the road. One of my native kidneys, even though it had had its wires disconnected, so to speak, had grown a huge stone. It was an invitation to a host of infections and needed to be removed urgently.

The doctors took the enlarged native kidney out: I bade farewell to dysfunctional Phinneas forever. Two weeks later, an exasperated me was back at Cedars-Sinai, yet again with elevated creatinine levels. It looked like it might be rejection. I spent December 31, 2005, in the hospital, getting doses of steroids. It was New Year's Eve. The ward was chillingly empty, working on a reduced staff. I saw the New Year in with a bowl of fat-free Very Vanilla Yoplait yogurt and graham crackers, an IV, and a suppository. Happy Friggin' New Year.

But after this sputtering start, my mother's kidney eventually stopped being mercurial and we became one. She calmed down and started working, just as I jumped back into the Hollywood fray in early 2006. Her creatinine numbers were gorgeous—or as my mother would say, *gorjus*—and together we were back eating McCarthy Salads at the Polo Lounge and enjoying prosperous health.

But in April of 2006, I was back in the hospital once more, and it wasn't her fault. After being cut open so many times, the organs in my abdomen were bulging out of their linings, a common complication of my kind of surgery. I had been sidelined by a hernia, which I tried to tell everyone was a sports injury from my days as the captain of the Notre Dame football team, but no one bought that story. After they sewed me up, I still spent almost a month in bed, motionless, recovering. My mother was once again my legs.

At the end of that month, I found myself driving to the hospital for another creatinine scare. Such is the life of a new transplantee: It takes a while for the kidney to function properly. It's not easy, or neat, the way a control freak like me would have liked it. It takes a while for the right med combination to do its work.

But this time I was released after my biopsy without any sign of rejection. Who knew what the future might hold, but for now, it looked like my mother's kidney had finally, happily, settled into my body for good. I retrieved my car from the Cedars-Sinai valet, pulled away from the parking lot, and didn't need to look in the rearview mirror.

CHAPTER 16

From Paris with Love

Depression doesn't send you a press release. It doesn't send you a reminder E-mail. You often have no idea when you're in it. I had no idea that the hardest part of my disease, the most devastating emotional fallout, would come when I was finally healthy. It took months after my return to normal life to understand why, when I should be happy, I felt so awful.

I went back to work full time on January 3, 2006, just two days after my New Year's biopsy slumber party at Cedars-Sinai. Awards season was weeks away, and I wasn't about to miss another red carpet, even if I had to wear a catheter and all of the regalia attached to it and stuff it into a YSL tuxedo. I was still bloated and drugged and crazy on steroids, but I was like a spotlight-craving diva who believes that the show must go on even if you have an ice pick in your neck. After being in and out of the hospital for a year, I wanted to be seen.

Plotting my return meant a major beauty tune-up. Rodeo Drive and the surrounding streets were shut down as every top skin technician, facialist, and scalp analyst in town converged to polish me to a high shine. In between twice-weekly blood tests to monitor my creatinine levels, the epogen shots to manage my ongoing anemia, the regular visits with Dr. Jordan and the trips to the drugstore to pick up bags stuffed with bottles of pills, I club-soda'd my way through every premiere in town and reacclimated myself to the art of party calisthenics: Jumping across the room to "accidentally" bump into über agent Kevin Huvane while simultaneously IMing Judd Apatow at the bar.

My agenda was simple: I had finally gotten the sickness "out of the way" and now it was time for yet another glorious comeback. I had convinced myself that the disease was all done, there would be no more side effects. I was going to forget that I'd ever been ill and prove to myself—and the world at large—that I was fine.

But it doesn't work like that. Disease doesn't just go away, even when it's gone.

The Golden Globes, broadcast on January 16, was the first event of the season, and I saw it as a litmus test. I was now back full time, after the long laundry list of things I'd been through the previous year, and I was finally stable. Unlike my "comeback" number one, the previous summer at the MTV VMAs, this return was no longer an innocent fantasy out of *Sunset Boulevard*. I felt more fragile: After being sliced and diced and pureed, would I even be able to stand up? Or was I just a shell of myself?

I also struggled with echoes of high-school paranoia about being accepted. After the first transplant, people had been generous; but after the second, would I be relegated to the graveyard? Did I really bring something to the red carpet or had my moment passed? I was feeling insecure, and I needed validation big time.

I walked onto the red carpet looking like a hot pocket in a tux. I climbed up on the *Entertainment Tonight* platform, and looked down at the air-kissing celebrities below me. I felt someone tapping on my foot: I glanced down to see George Clooney, smiling up at me with his million-watt grin. "How are you feeling, Cojo?" he asked, with warm genuine eyes. "Are you OK?"

"Actually, my doctor says that I'm going to kick the bucket unless

I shack up with you at your villa on the restorative waters of Lake Como."

"Sure," he said. "Anytime. Just as long as I'm not there."

The next weeks were a blur of sun-damaged cleavage, starched hair, and sweat-stained chiffon. Awards season in Hollywood runs about the course of a staph infection: A two-month marathon where the featured dish at every fete is ego l'orange and baked bullshit Alaska for dessert. Like a starved starlet fallen off the carb-free wagon, I feasted on both dishes at the SAG awards, the Grammy awards, the Oscars, and every pre-, post-, and in-between party in town.

There was certainly no room in my day planner for introspection. And yet, as awards season wore on, I found myself feeling empty and questioning the meaning of everything I saw around me. At first, sheer adrenaline kept me going, but now I was starting to crack. Physically, I was exhausted: My body hadn't yet healed, and I was tired, in pain, constantly short of breath. What once had been so easy now felt like too much work. I wasn't the same person anymore; not physically, not emotionally. The world and the job that I once wore so comfortably, like a fine cashmere coat, felt off.

By the time the Grammy's rolled around at the end of February, I was on the verge of collapse. The day of the event, I woke up without the slightest excitement about going—and for me to lose interest in dishing with Fergie on the red carpet is a very big deal indeed. That night, I did my interviews on the red carpet with only perfunctory enthusiasm, barely able to muster interest in the stampede of Gwen Stefani's giddy Harajuku girls, and fled back home as soon as the red carpet was being dismantled.

As soon as I walked in the door of my house, I collapsed. My BlackBerry was vibrating. My cell phone said that there were twenty-seven messages. I ignored them all: I took my antirejection pills, grabbed my dog, kicked my boots off, and collapsed on the living room couch. I hugged Stinky close to my chest, feeling engulfed by some undefinable malaise. What was wrong with me? I should be *celebrating*, not feeling so down.

Any other time, I would be busy conducting my post–award show ritual. First, I would neurotically put away my wardrobe by steaming the wrinkles out of my suit and hermetically seal it in a garment bag. I would then fold every other item (including socks) and put them away, too. I would then go through a rigorous drill of makeup re-moval using four cleansers, sandpaper, and Lysol disinfectant wipes. Not that night. I couldn't muster the energy. I just collapsed on the couch in full stage makeup, still dressed in my Grammy regalia. I woke up hours later, with crusty mascara smeared all over my white couch and my white dog, my satin suit crinkled into origami.

I sunk even further when I woke up the following day. Not even a shot of pomegranate juice with bee pollen could lift me from my funk. I skipped my business meetings, missed my blood test ap-pointment at the clinic, and just slept. I did all my work by E-mail, incapable of even speaking on the phone. Prone in my bed, I couldn't understand what was wrong with me.

But the feeling pervaded as the days passed. Mostly, I felt tre-mendously lost. For the first time in over a year, I didn't have people holding my hand and coddling me: My parents and Shari had long ago returned to Canada, I wasn't being monitored hourly by a troop of nurses and doctors, and my friends no longer were obliged to call and check in on me every day. Because I was healthy now, it also meant that I had to fend for myself.

New emotional anxieties assaulted me every day, a laundry list of things to be paranoid about: I panicked about forgetting to take those pills, worried about the kidney rejecting, obsessed over the feeling that I was permanently handicapped. I wasn't like other people, anymore: I was separated by my experience.

Awards season marched on. I had to be upbeat and energetic, despite feeling like I was sinking in quicksand. All through February and March I kept up the illusion, until the very last celebrity had departed the Oscars Governor's Ball and bundled their rumpled couture into their limousines.

But back at home, I would fall apart. Nothing could comfort me. All my crutches were gone, nary a vice. Even though I had a clean bill of health, there was no drinking, no carousing, no inhaling. I was even forced to throw away the bong made of Moroccan glass that Snoop Dogg had given me as a Chanukah present. Instead, the only panacea was sleep.

I was consumed by napping: I considered every other activity an interruption. Life became like marking things off a to-do list so I could climb back into bed. I would go on sleep benders, sleeping days at a time, with the curtains drawn and the room blacked out. It was hot out: I pumped the air-conditioning on its most frigid setting, just so I could curl up under three comforters. I liked my depression on ice: The room echoed how I felt, undeserving of fresh air and sunlight.

Making a meal was a task as monumental as building a skyscraper. My kitchen was abandoned: The desire to sleep was stronger than the hunger pangs. I took hour-long showers, hoping that the hot water would wash off this gray film of bleakness. I turned on my beloved Stinky: I resented having to take care of another creature. Sometimes his morning walk wouldn't happen until noon. I would wake up at 7:00 a.m. and start sending signals to my brain that Stinky needed to be taken out. But then I would turn over, go back to sleep. For the next six hours I would drift in and out of consciousness, as the signals warned me *Take him out! Take him out!* Stinky would lie next to me, whimpering; and yet I still couldn't summon the will to do it. I got to a place where I didn't care if he made in the bed—or even if I did.

I visited a therapist. "What are you here to talk about?" he asked.

"I had a medical tragedy last year, and now I'm having a really hard time coping with life." I explained to him. "It feels like it's all too much."

He took notes and nodded. I waited for him to give me answers that would solve my problems, but he just stared at me, letting me babble incessantly. I left the office feeling gypped: He didn't give me anything useful; he didn't give me a plan. I wanted to quickly fix the pain and lift this depression, and I wanted to do it *now*. I was too new to therapy to realize there was true work involved. I simply didn't show up to our next appointment.

Like speed-dating, I went through a slew of buttoned-up PhDs before I finally found a therapist who I connected with. I had finally found someone with whom communication was easy, and it felt like we were working together. I didn't feel alone anymore: Someone finally understood and felt empathetic. My post-recovery depression, my therapist told me, was a common complaint of disease survivors: The real pain comes afterward, when you go back to your life. Since the summer of 2004, I had been dealt blow after blow, but I was too busy surviving—living from blood test to blood test, creatinine number to creatinine number—and I simply hadn't had the room in my overloaded psyche to process the real trauma of my disease. Instead, I'd buried my emotions, and now they were coming back to bite me.

In March of 2007, my kidney took its first transatlantic flight. I'd landed in Paris. I had my dream itinerary in my hands, the one I'd been imagining since I lay half-dead, defeated, in the dialysis center. It was the grand finale of my personal kidney movie, and I wasn't solo: It was a trip for two, me and my spiffy new kidney.

It was an enchanted week. We visited the tearoom above the Ladurée patisserie and indulged in the same *chocolat amer macarons* that Marie Antoinette had satisfied her sweet tooth with. I salivated over vintage Chanel jewelry at a secret boutique hidden on a side street on the Left Bank, fondling original brooches that Coco herself had once worn. We finished our evening with a special date at the illuminated Opéra, where we stood outside in a light rain and absorbed the facade as if it were a painting: When the Opéra is glowing in the rain, it almost seems divine.

Our weeklong tour came to an end at my favorite spot in Paris: The Tuileries garden at twilight, where I sat by my favorite fountain. This was supposed to be the moment where the soundtrack swells up: After all the strife I'd been through, my magical city and my magical spot was going to finally give me the big epiphany I needed for closure . . . the happy ending. But where was it?

Nearly a year had passed since my last overnight stay at Cedars-Sinai. I hadn't suddenly lifted out of my depression: There was no magic formula. I couldn't define the single event that had made me feel better. Instead, I had clocked in a lot of time in therapy, slowly dealing with emotion head on. All my life, I had kept my feelings bottled up inside—the lifelong scars and past rejections, the pent-up anger and low self-esteem—but this seminal event in my life had crashed my emotional system and now I had to rethink everything.

I had to learn to deal not just with the aftermath of my disease, but take emotional stock of a life's worth of baggage.

There were days when I felt so cold and emotionless that it was as if my heart had turned into granite. Other days, I was filled with fury. And sometimes, the wind would blow in another bout of depression. But now I knew what that monster was. It was a matter of using all my strength to pull myself out of bed and use the skills I'd learned in therapy to march forward instead of hiding under the covers.

But I still didn't have a life. That was the surprise discovery of my year-long recovery. I had woken up one morning with this horrifying, palpitating realization: I had a career, I had a wardrobe alphabetized by designer label, I had a freshly detailed sports car. But a life? No. All these years, I had been such a driven animal, so blinded by my career, that I wasn't aware that my whole life was about my job. I had spent half my life on an airplane. I was like a vampire, only slithering out at night. All I did was work work work. Once I had passed through the worst of my illness, I didn't know what to do with myself. After all I'd worked for, I didn't know how to do anything besides take celebrities to task for their fashion faux pas and showcase my own snappy ensembles. The joke was on me.

But now I was actually learning how to have a life again. How to make time for friends. How to invite people to hang out at home in sweatpants. How to go through an entire meal without once mentioning show business or fashion. I wanted to stop and smell the patchouli candles. I was in training. Already, I was starting to consider new hobbies. Songwriting, baking devil's food cupcakes, skeet shooting, elementary monster truck driving. Expressionist painting. Bead making. Growing hemp. Harp classes. I was even getting in touch with my paternal instincts: Dressing Stinky up in Baby Dior outfits and teaching him French.

Sitting there in the Tuileries gardens, I thought of my mother, and how much she had wanted this trip for me. That, I realized, was the other surprise to come out of my illness: Looking back now, I knew that as terrible as the last few years had been, they had also brought my family closer together. Suffering together had turned us into a strong unit. After going through all our travails, we could look at each other now and ask ourselves, what's worth fighting about? We were proud of ourselves: This is who we are. This is our family.

It started to get cold in this peaceful garden. I shivered. There would be no Hollywood-ending sunset tonight, no snapshot moment to end my Paris vacation, but it didn't matter to me anymore. Life is not a movie, I realized. Life was not the postcards I'd always painted in my head. Unlike the movie star that I'd always been in my own mind, the real me was flawed. Sometimes even a mess. But maybe that was OK. Maybe having my life turned upside down turned out to be the healing that I needed: I didn't have to live up to my own picture-perfect expectations anymore. It didn't matter what I didn't have. Whatever I had *was* enough, because I was alive.

Learn More About Kidney Disease

More than 20 million people in America live with chronic kidney disease. At any given moment, roughly 63,000 patients are on a waiting list for a kidney transplant: The demand for organs drastically exceeds the number that are available for transplant. As a result, some patients will die before they ever locate a new kidney.

By becoming a living donor, you can make a real difference in a kidney disease patient's life. Transplants that come from living donors are more likely to work right away, and less likely to be rejected.

If you have a friend or family member who is looking for a kidney transplant—or even wish to donate an organ to a stranger in need—consider becoming a living donor. Talk to your doctor, or call the National Kidney Foundation at 1-800-622-9010.

For more information about organ donation, visit the following Web sites:

National Kidney Foundation's Living Donors Online

www.livingdonors.org

Transplant Living

www.transplantliving.org

United Network for Organ Sharing

www.unos.org/data/about/viewDataReports.asp

Acknowledgments

Dr. Stanley Jordan, a truly awe-inspiring man of greatness. I am so blessed to have someone as compassionate, caring, and dedicated as you in my life.

Dr. Louis J. Cohen, surgeon extraordinaire and kind therapist to my parents. Here's to your lifetime supply of Cristal.

Robin Hudson, the best hand-holder in the world. Thank you for always wearing a nice cheerful lip stain before my surgeries.

The kidney clinic team at Cedars-Sinai who enveloped me in warmth and love. You are the angels who carried me through.

All the incredibly kind nurses at Cedars-Sinai who let me pass the time by giving you makeovers.

All my love and gratitude to Shari Isenberg for your absolute devotion and for wearing lipstick so bright I could find my morphine drip button in the dark.

Linda and Steve Levine, thank you for always being my safety net.

Linda Bell Blue, Terry Wood, and Janet Annino, thank you for pushing me to excel and be better, and for being there with open arms when I fell.

Special thanks to Sandi Mendelson, Paul Olsewski, Judy Hilsinger, and Scott "Margaritaville" Zolke.

My literary agent Jay Mandel; this is our second book together—I think we now have the formula—just make them entirely about me.

And to my editor Kathy Huck, thank you for believing and standing by this book. It's as much yours as it is mine.